THE FOOD QUESTION

THE FOOD QUESTION

VARIOUS

ISBN: 978-93-89614-32-9

Published: -

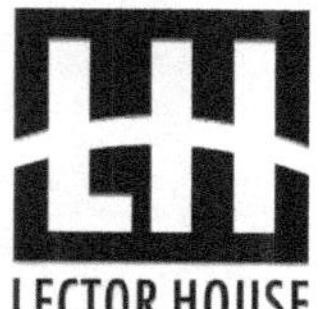

LECTOR HOUSE LLP
E-MAIL: lectorpublishing@gmail.com

THE FOOD QUESTION
HEALTH AND ECONOMY

BY

EIGHT SPECIALISTS

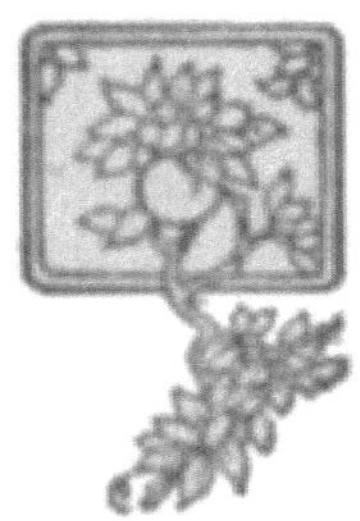

"Eat ye that which is good."
"That thou mayest prosper and be in health."
"Eat in due season, for strength, and not for drunkenness."
"Gather up the fragments that remain, that nothing be lost."

LELAND STANFORD JUNIOR UNIVERSITY

OFFICE OF THE PRESIDENT

Stanford University, California.

10 Oct. '17

Mr. N. C. Wilcox,
Mountain View, Cal.

Dear Mr. Wilcox,

May I thank you for your kindness in sending me proofs of your food question Book, which I have gone over with much interest. It is very gratifying to note that the general plan recommended by you fits so well into the suggestions of the Food Administration.

The great necessity is to teach our people the use of the various substitute foods, which we have in abundance and thereby save the wheat, meat, pork produce, dairy products, and sugar required to meet the needs of our allies and to supply the deficiencies in the neutral countries. Every step that can be taken in the education of our people along these lines is a service, not only to the nations, but also to humanity in general. With our surplus food stocks, the problem is a difficult one and a test of our intelligence, our far-sightedness, as well as of our patriotism and our humanity.

Very truly yours,

Dr. Ray Lyman Wilbur
President.

PUBLISHERS' FOREWORD

This book was planned before Food Conservation was by the mass considered seriously. The writers of the various articles are thoroughly qualified to speak where they have spoken. They are practical, conscientious, Christian, and have at heart the best in the needs of humanity. Every one strikes a major chord in the song of healthful, economical living. The recipes are from the author of "Food and Cookery," who has had a score of years' experience in every station and phase of the preparation of food, under French, English, German, and Spanish chefs. He has been second cook in the Calumet Club of Chicago, the California Club, Los Angeles, and in many leading hotels in various cities. For ten years, he has given his best thought and study to the preparation of the best in food, scientific, palatable, wholesome, and economic, most of this time in the Sanitarium and College of Medical Missionaries, Loma Linda, California. Special attention is called to the valuable tables of Food Elements, and to the newly demonstrated values of vitamines and the substances which destroy them.

We are grateful for the kind word spoken by Dr. Ray Lyman Wilbur, president of Stanford University, and first assistant to Mr. Hoover in the Federal Food Administration Department; also for the help and suggestions of Dr. Newton Evans, president of the College of Medical Evangelists, of Loma Linda, California.

The little book will, we believe, not only meet present needs, but be a safe counselor in the years to come.

HOOVER SAYS— WILSON SAYS—

Hoover Says —

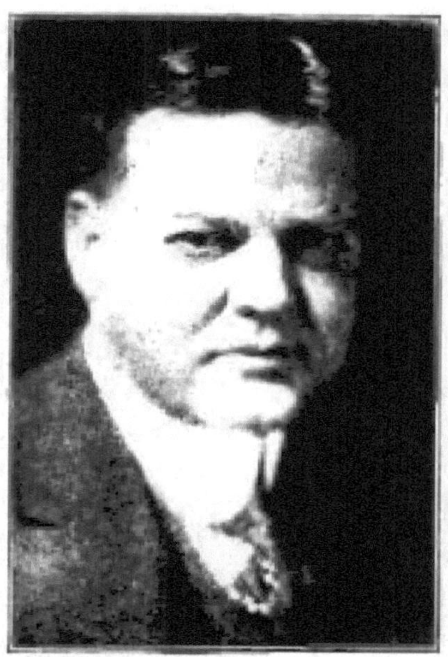

Hoover

"LET the American woman *s t o p* , before anything is thrown away; and let her ask herself, 'Can it be used in my home, in some other home, or in the production of further food supply by feeding it to animals used also for food?'

"Let her *o r d e r* her meals so that there will be plenty—for there is *p l e n - t y* —but not too much.

"The intelligent woman of America must make a proper study of food ratios, so that the most nutritious foods will appear in their proper proportions on the home table.

"The man who complains at the result of his wife's efforts to conserve food is doing her an inexcusable injury. He should never hesitate to coöperate in her wise conservation plans."

Wilson says —

"IN no direction can they [the women of America] so greatly assist as by enlisting in the service of the food administration and cheerfully accepting its direction and advice. By so doing, they will increase the surplus of food available for our own army and for exports to the allies. To provide adequate supplies for the coming year is of absolutely vital importance to the conduct of the war; and without a very conscientious elimination of waste and very strict economy in our food consumption, we cannot hope to fulfill this primary duty."

CONTENTS

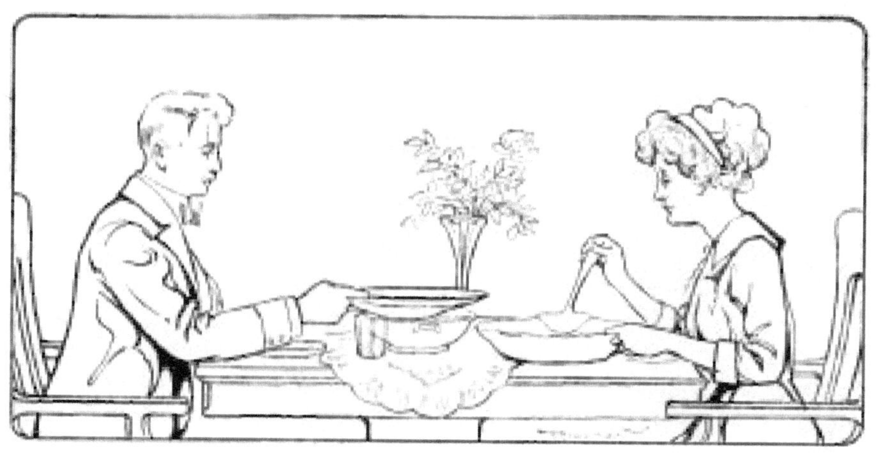

FOOD ECONOMY

BY
E. A. SUTHERLAND, A. B., M. D.

of the State Bureau of
Food Conservation of Tennessee

From the days of ancient Egypt, when Joseph, who stood at the head of the great food conservation movement of the time, called the attention of the world to the need of food economy, down through history to the present time, the human race has passed through numerous crises when the questions of food production and food economy have been vital. That Hebrew, promoted to the first place in the Egyptian empire because of his wonderful grasp of a world problem and his executive ability, enabled that kingdom to feed the world. America to-day, as Egypt of old, is an international granary, and is asked to feed the nations; and her population—every man, woman, and child—must coöperate with America's Joseph to-day in meeting the situation by proper production, proper conservation, and strict economy. "This war is a food war even more than it is a gun war." Let us fight to save lives. That is the battle to be won through food economy.

It was when the Roman world was running riot that, on the shores of the Sea of Galilee, Christ gave His wonderful lesson on the subject of food conservation. We call it a miracle when with five thousand men, besides the women and the children, seated about Him, He fed the multitudes. That same power is to-day, and always has been, feeding the men of earth. From a basket of seed, each recurring harvest puts thousands of loaves of bread into the hands of the world's hungry; the two small fishes continue to multiply; rich and poor alike are fed by the great Provider. And now as then, after human wants are met, the mandate goes forth,

"Gather up the fragments that remain, that nothing be lost." Economy is again being preached as it was once taught on the shores of Galilee. There has been started a great educational movement for increased food production. But that is only a part of the message. "Gather up the fragments," prevent waste, utilize the scraps, the gospel of a clean plate, — these are all familiar phrases in the great conservation movement of to-day. By many, food conservation and food economy are deemed not only national problems, but a part of the divine message taught by Christ and His disciples.

The great world war which began in 1914 has compelled every nation to halt and consider its national habits.

Undoubtedly the United States is the most prodigal of nations. Approximately sixty per cent of its population is now urban. Simple rural life is practically gone; and those artificial and extravagant standards of the city which destroy body, mind, and soul have taken its place. "Fullness of bread and abundance of idleness," two of the reasons assigned by the Scriptures for the downfall of Sodom, are conditions which to-day are ruining American civilization. No other nation has ever indulged such extravagance and prodigality as has the United States. We search the world over for table delicacies. American inventive genius has made it possible to have foods from all parts of the world, both in season and out of season. The arts of canning and preserving and the making of factory foods have loaded our cupboard shelves with eatables of which our fathers never dreamed.

While this interchange has its advantages, and we should appreciate the privilege of eating the wholesome products of other countries, yet when easy methods of transportation lead people to limit their productions to money crops, forsaking the raising of their own food, a wrong principle has been introduced. The benefit to be derived from this variety of imported food is neutralized by the extravagant habits and tastes thus cultivated.

Economy of Food Elements

Man is made from the dust of the earth; and by divine law, his body continues to build and rebuild from chemically organized soil. To be intelligent, food economists require a knowledge of the four food elements, — proteins, carbohydrates, fats, and minerals, — and the relation each sustains to the human body. Later chapters contain valuable instruction in these respects.

It is poor economy to allow valuable mineral salts to be removed from flour by milling, from rice by polishing, and from vegetables by wrong methods of cooking. These minerals are necessary for the development of the child, for the preservation of teeth and bones, for high efficiency in the nervous system, and for a proper functioning of the various organs in the body. There is no economy in buying denatured grain, even though it is put up in cartons, at ten times the price of the natural grain.

"Put a knife to thy throat, if thou be a man given to appetite." Stop the immense waste of strength, energy, money, and time due to mere gratification of appetite. Stop preparing food that is intended simply to coax the appetite to the point where eating becomes gluttony. In the words of an eminent authority, "Most men would attain better health and greater efficiency if they would reduce their rations by twenty-five per cent or more." The celebrated Dr. Osler tells us that "we eat too much after forty years of age," and he advises every wise man to restrict his eating as he grows older, "and at last descend out of life as he ascended into it, even into a child's diet."

Overeating

Food economy is not a call to a starvation diet, but to a balanced ration of wholesome, well prepared food. Overeating of even the best food produces poisons that injure the tissues, overwork the organs of digestion, and in time may bring the body to actual starvation conditions.

A man's appetite is not always a safe guide. Artificial surroundings in childhood make the normal appetite the exception rather than the rule. Few children are taught, by parents, teachers, or preachers, the importance of restricting the appetite. The seeds of intemperance sown by those who prepare food for the family table bring a larger harvest than does the work of all the devil's agencies in saloons and tobacco shops combined. Millions of dollars are worse than wasted by the conversion of food materials into strong drinks to satisfy appetites perverted by wrong habits of eating. Why are our schools and churches more interested in the maintenance of a worn-out, traditional educational system, and an abstract, impractical religion, than in some of these vital teachings? We look to legislation to cure degenerate appetites for which we are largely responsible through false education in home and school and church. Starving ones of earth are deprived of food when we convert it into strong drink; the process requires the time and strength of a great army of workers; and transportation facilities now used for carrying whisky, tobacco, and other body- and mind-destroying substances, might be used in transporting the foods we waste. It is estimated that we waste enough in our kitchens to feed ten million people. "Blessed art thou, O land, when ... thy princes eat in due season, for strength, and not for drunkenness!"

Some Economies

Dr. Osler has said that "pie north of the Mason and Dixon line, and hot bread south of it, have done more harm than alcohol." The best breads contain the whole grain; they are well baked, require considerable chewing, resist the pressure of the teeth, and save dental bills. Thorough mastication neutralizes an abnormal appetite.

Rich pastries, harmful condiments, tea and coffee,—narcotics recognized as extravagant, harmful, and useless beverages,—are being discarded for the sake of both health and economy. Remove the cream and the sugar from tea and coffee, and they have no food value.

Use the coffee mill to grind wheat, rye, and corn, that you may enjoy the vitamines, the mineral salts, and other elements often removed by the manufacturer.

Many people prominent in social circles are eliminating all lunches served between regular meals and eaten for merely social purposes. Such lunches impose a burden on the body and the purse. Wealthy and influential women are setting a good example by going to market in person, in order to make intelligent and economical purchases for their tables, and by carrying their supplies home, in order to save the added cost of the delivery system. People are beginning to realize that by such economical methods, they can serve their country, the world, and themselves.

Some have thought it necessary to eat from three to five meals a day. The war is helping them to appreciate a physiological truth taught for years by a few reformers,—that two meals a day are better even than three.

Many countries, for economy's sake, now prohibit the use, for food, of young and undeveloped animals. They discourage the extensive use of immature plant foods. The world war is terrible, yet there is some compensation in the fact that present conditions are making minds more susceptible to the principles of right living. For years, some earnest men and women have been teaching that God intended that man should live on a meatless diet. To-day, not only are nations asking that men eat less meat, but they are having their meatless days. Because of the impossibility of securing flesh foods in some countries, millions of earth's inhabitants have learned that the body can be kept in splendid condition without the use of animal proteins and fats. No strong arguments are necessary to convince people that flesh foods are expensive when it is known that ten pounds of grain suitable for human food are required to produce in the animal one pound of flesh food.

Meat Substitutes

The high cost of flesh foods is turning attention to meat substitutes. Proteins and fats of the vegetable world are not only cheaper, but they are more wholesome than flesh. For example: The soy bean, recently introduced to the American table, contains, pound for pound, and at one fifth the cost, almost twice as much available protein and fat as the best beefsteak. Besides that, it offers the eater a good supply of starch.

"We have got to learn to buy wisely, cook wisely, eat wisely, and waste nothing." The great countries of Europe are utilizing the best talent of their statesmen and scientists in teaching the people these ideas. This should be a most impressive lesson to home, to church, and to school, since these agencies have so far forgotten their mission that it is necessary for this great war to arouse us.

Let religious and educational leaders redeem the time. Let them coöperate with national economists who now are urging the people—

To use more home-ground flour and meal.

To use the natural rice with its vitamines instead of the polished product.

To substitute vegetable oils for dairy butter in cooking.

To have a simpler variety of food at each meal.

To serve a dessert, when one is deemed necessary, for its food value and as a part of a balanced ration.

To bake or boil potatoes in the skins, in order to preserve the mineral salts.

To utilize for soups and gravies the water in which vegetables, macaroni, and rice are boiled.

To serve only one food of high protein value at a meal.

To feed to animals nothing that can be utilized by the human body.

To allow vegetables, grains, and legumes to ripen, that their full food value may be obtained, and that the expense of canning may be avoided.

To can or dry all fruits and vegetables that cannot be preserved in any other way.

To substitute other cereals for wheat, which can be shipped abroad.

A wheatless meal every day will drive many to appreciate the value of other grains, whose use heretofore has been largely perverted. Corn, rye, barley, and oats are not appreciated as they should be. They have been used largely in the manufacture of intoxicating drinks and for feeding animals to procure meat. It has been said that the Revolutionary War was won by men fed on hasty pudding — in other words, corn meal mush. Learn to eat bread made from corn, rye, or oats, or a mixture of these grains. Form the habit of eating these more economical breads; then continue the practice. Such breads are far superior to the ordinary denatured white bread. If a dog is fed only white bread, death will result sooner than if it is fed nothing.

The Call of the Country

Land in Europe that for centuries was used to gratify the abnormal tastes of plutocrats and the aristocracy, is now being made to produce wholesome food to meet the world's needs. In America, people are still deprived of their divine right to a simple home, because millions of acres of land are held in a similar manner.

Schools and churches should encourage the cultivation of vacant city lots. City people may thus learn the secret of intensive farming. It may give some courage to make a home on a few acres of land and to raise the food for their own tables. Every turn in a congested center calls for an outlay of means. Modern methods of living are unnatural and extravagant. In the city, every article of food costs in proportion to its distance from the base of supplies. Transportation must be added to the original cost of production; the jobber, the wholesaler, the commission merchant, the retailer, the delivery man, and the baker must all have their profits.

Get out of the cities; get onto the land! Why not preach this part of the gospel? Help people to understand that the unnatural appetites and the desires for artificial food are penalties paid very largely by those who seek to maintain themselves by their wits. One mighty step has been taken toward the prevention of waste and in economy's favor when men learn to earn their bread in the sweat of their face while tilling the soil.

Late hours, business worry, nerve-wrecking noises, the hurry, the wear and tear of living in a crowd, the dust and filth of the city air, the struggle of competition,—these would be replaced by purer, saner surroundings if parents settled in some country place where children are born with a heritage of fresh air, grassy playgrounds, wholesome daily tasks in the house and out of doors, and are fed in a simple manner befitting their surroundings. But do not transfer the evils of the city to some country site. Not much need to urge "the gospel of the clean plate" to the healthy country child! A good appetite is the best seasoning for plain food.

Permanent Reforms

The world has been roughly awakened, and forcibly compelled to study food economy. This upheaval should result in permanent good to every individual. We have not fully appreciated the fact that our sinful indulgence and our careless waste of time, money, and food is a violation of the great commandment, "Thou shalt love thy neighbor as thyself." By our extravagant ways, multitudes have been robbed of the necessities of life. But our horizon is broadening. We begin to understand why we should eat and drink to the glory of God. Provision is now being made for the bread we save to reach the hungry in distant parts of the earth. We can now prove that he who gives even a cup of cold water shall in no wise lose his reward. To-day, as truly as on the shores of Galilee, the great Master is saying, "Gather up the fragments that remain, that nothing be lost." And if we enter whole-heartedly into this food conservation movement, we may expect the blessing of the Lord to rest so greatly upon the fragments saved that the wide world will be fed.

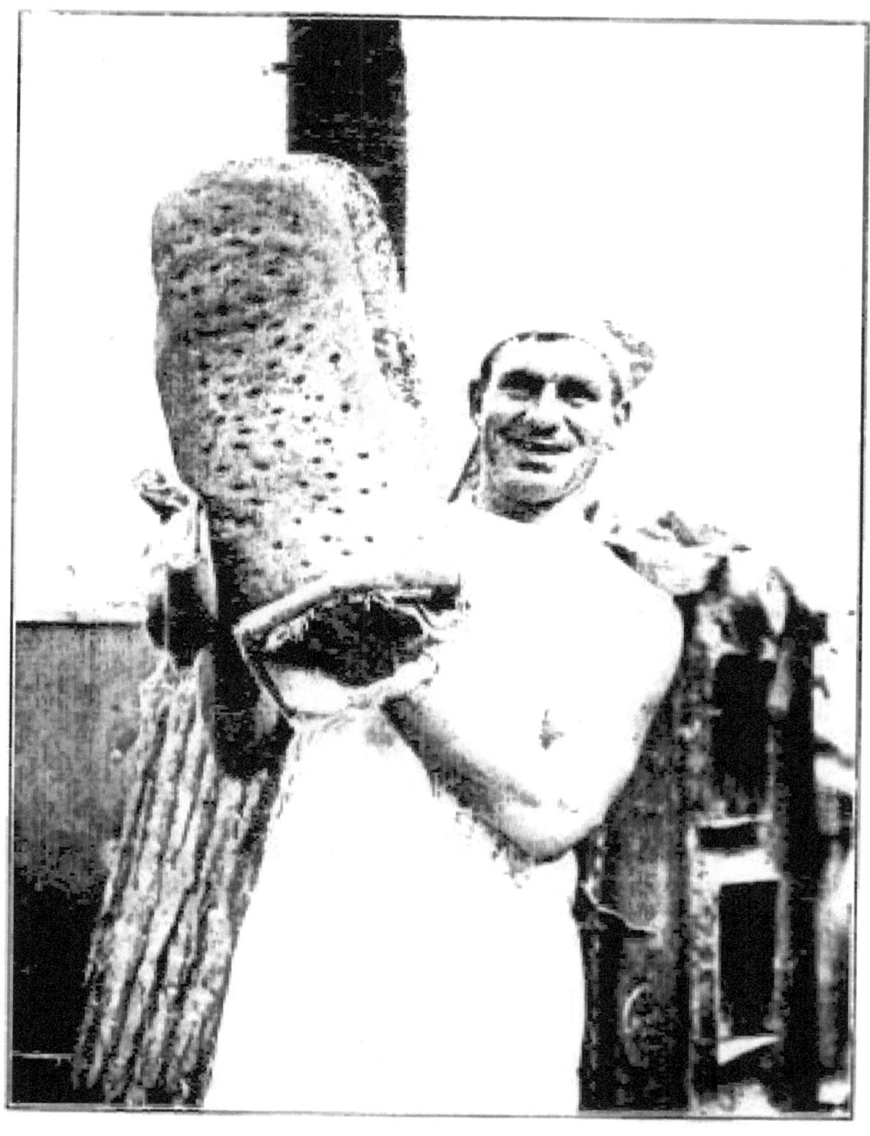

© Underwood, N. Y.

A ten-pound loaf of war bread baked on the old Gettysburg battle field. This bread keeps in good condition three weeks.

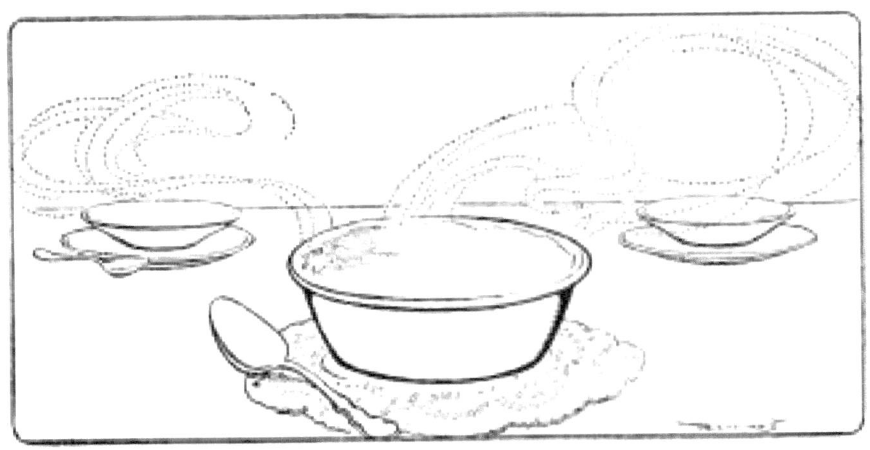

FOOD ELEMENTS AND SIMPLICITY OF DIET

BY
E. H. RISLEY, M.D.

Chair of Chemistry, College of Medical Evangelists,
Loma Linda, California

"Food is any substance that, being taken into the body of animal or plant, serves, through organic action, to build up normal structure or supply waste of tissue."

Food principles or elements are commonly grouped into the following classes:

- 1. Proteins
- 2. Fats
- 3. Carbohydrates
- 4. Inorganic salts
- 5. Vitamines
- 6. Water

A brief discussion of these food elements will help our readers to select their food supply more intelligently.

Proteins

The first class of food substances mentioned above are of very great importance to the body. The term "protein" really means, "of first importance." These compounds are represented by such foods as the white of egg, lean meat, gluten of wheat, and casein of milk. Chemically, proteins are very complex, more so than any other class of food materials. They have in their structure the chemical elements carbon, hydrogen, oxygen, nitrogen, often sulphur and phosphorus, and, less commonly, iron. The nitrogenous element seems to be the most important, since the others mentioned can be obtained from other classes of food; but as these classes of food cannot take the place of protein, it seems clear that the nitrogen is the important constituent.

Most proteins coagulate on heating. An illustration of this property is the coagulation of the white of an egg when the egg is cooked. The proteins all undergo decomposition quite easily. This is evidenced by the ease with which eggs and meat spoil.

Protein molecules are made up of smaller molecules called amino acids. These are the "building stones" from which the working tissues of the body are formed. There are on the average about fifteen different kinds of these amino acids in the proteins, which are especially valuable in supplying building material for the tissues of the human body. These amino acids are united in long chains to form the protein molecule, and in this respect can be compared to cars in a train. By the work of digestion, the proteins are broken down into these comparatively simple building stones, which, when absorbed into the circulation, are used by the body in building working tissues as they are needed.

There are a number of classes of proteins; but since the classification is rather complicated, it will not be given here. To group the various foods as to their relative amounts of protein is often of interest. For example, foods very rich in protein, such as the gluten preparations, lean beef, and white of egg, may be regarded as the first class; a second class might be formed of those which are moderately high in protein, such as peas, beans, lentils, and walnuts; a third class having a moderate amount of protein, represented by the cereals and breads; and still a fourth class very low in protein, such as vegetables and fruits.

Protein is the tissue builder of the body; but the actual amount of tissue built new each day is very small, therefore the need for a large supply of protein for this purpose is not apparent. Protein not only supplies tissue-building material, but it can also supply heat and energy in a manner similar to the other classes of food elements, carbohydrate and fat, one ounce of the protein yielding one hundred sixteen calories of energy. The excess taken in may be used in this way, as there is no storage of this material in the body. However, to use this kind of fuel takes more work on the part of the body as a whole, as the nitrogenous wastes must be eliminated by the kidneys.

One can see, then, that a certain amount of protein is needed to keep the tissues in good repair, but that it is better to get most of the heat and energy from the food elements specially designed for that purpose; that is, carbohydrate and fat.

The Chittenden standard of diet gives ten per cent of the total fuel value in the form of protein. On the basis of two thousand five hundred total calories a day, two hundred fifty calories of protein would be required. This is equal to two and one seventh ounces actual dry protein. This amount is thought by some to be low, but experimental evidence seems clearly to prove its adequacy in keeping up nutrition.

Fats

The second group of food elements in our classification are substances having a greasy feeling and taste. They are lighter than water, leave a grease spot upon paper, are insoluble in water, and soluble in such chemicals as gasoline and ether.

Fats have in their molecules the chemical elements carbon, hydrogen, and oxygen. These elements are put together into two groups, or compounds, glycerin and fatty acids, which, when chemically united, form a fat. When fats are exposed to the open air, and thus contaminated with bacteria, they are likely to become rancid; that is, some of the glycerin and fatty acids are set free from each other. If butter is the fat so decomposed, it becomes very disagreeable, on account of the volatile butyric acid that is set free.

Fatty bodies are usually grouped under a general heading called lipins, but the consideration of the other classes is not essential in this study.

The vegetable kingdom offers a large list of products containing fats, many of which are suitable for food. Following are a few examples, with the percentage of fat in each case: coconuts, sixty-eight per cent; olives, fifty-six per cent; peanuts, forty-one per cent; cotton seed, twenty per cent; oatmeal, six per cent; corn, four per cent.

The animal kingdom is also rich in fat products, illustrated by the following substances used as foods: butter, eighty-five per cent; bacon, sixty-five per cent; cheese, thirty per cent; eggs, eleven per cent; cow's milk, four per cent.

The function of fat in the body is to yield heat and energy primarily. Each ounce of fat yields two hundred sixty-four calories of heat, making the group two and one fourth times as active as either protein or carbohydrate in this respect.

Fats ordinarily supply from twenty-five to thirty per cent of the total calories of a well balanced dietary. On the basis of two thousand five hundred total calories a day, about seven hundred fifty should be fat. At two hundred sixty-four calories to an ounce, we have about three ounces as our daily need of this food element.

Fats are also stored in the body as a reserve of energy. Every one has more or less of this sort of reserve, unless he has been starving for some time, or is suffering from a wasting disease. This reserve of fat also acts as a protection, and gives shape and symmetry to the body.

Recently methods have been devised for changing the unstable vegetable oils into stable, lardlike, solid fats. This process is called hydrogenation, so named because the process is really one of adding hydrogen until the fat becomes saturated and less likely to undergo decomposition into fatty acid and glycerin. The fats thus formed seem to be equal to the animal fats so far as digestion and utilization are concerned, and hence are of considerable economic value at the present time.

Certain fats, including those of butter and milk, are rich in the so-called vitamines, and have been shown, by recent experiments upon animals, to be efficient growth stimulants.

Carbohydrates

The carbohydrates are made up of the chemical elements carbon, hydrogen, and oxygen. By noticing the name, one readily sees that the first part stands for the carbon. The latter half, "hydrate," indicates that water might be present; and in fact, nearly all of these bodies have hydrogen and oxygen present in the proportion to form water, that is, two parts hydrogen to one of oxygen. Carbohydrates ordinarily make up about sixty to sixty-five per cent of the total number of calories of our diet. Most carbohydrates, when pure, are either white powders or white crystalline solids. Many of them are sweet to the taste. The starches and the celluloses are not soluble in cold water, but the sugars are readily soluble.

The classification of the carbohydrates is comparatively simple; and part of it is given here, as it will help in our discussion of the properties of the group:

Carbohydrates	1. Starch Group	1. Cellulose 2. Starch 3. Dextrin
	2. Cane Sugar Group	1. Cane Sugar 2. Malt Sugar 3. Milk Sugar
	3. Glucose Group	1. Glucose 2. Levulose 3. Invert Sugar

Cellulose is the coarse woody fiber found in the stems of all plants and in the outer coating of the various grains. Unless cellulose is very young and tender, it is not digested by the human digestive system. However, some forms of it are of value, as they give bulk to the food residue in the digestive tract, and thus stimulate the activity of the intestinal muscle. In this way, cellulose acts as a natural laxative, and in some cases is a very desirable substance to have in the food eaten. The bran of wheat and other cereals is an especially valuable form to use.

Starch is found in all cereals, in many vegetables, in some fruits, and in nuts. It occurs in these different foods in the form of a white, granular substance. The granules have characteristic forms for the different grains, fruits, etc., which can be recognized by the aid of the microscope. Raw starch is insoluble in cold water; hence to be most readily digested, it should be cooked. The cooking process ruptures the granules, and makes the starch itself partially soluble; and in this form, it is more easily attacked by the digestive juices.

Dextrin is formed by heating starch to about 350° F., as in an oven. This degree of heat changes the starch chemically to dextrin. In this dextrin form, it is soluble, and is in reality one step along in the process of digestion.

TABLE A—CEREALS AND LEGUMES

A. Per cent Water
B. Per cent Protein

C. Per cent Fat	
D. Per cent Carbohydrate	
E. Per cent Ash	
F. Calories per oz. Protein	
G. Calories per oz. Fat	
H. Calories per oz. Carbohydrate	
I. Calories per oz. Total	

FOOD	A	B	C	D	E	F	G	H	I
Beans, baked	68.9	6.9	2.5	19.6	2.1	8.0	6.6	22.7	37.3
Bread, white	35.3	9.2	1.3	53.1	1.1	10.7	3.4	61.6	75.7
Bread, whole wheat	38.4	9.7	.9	49.7	1.3	11.3	2.4	57.7	71.4
Corn bread	38.9	7.9	4.7	46.3	2.2	9.2	12.4	53.7	75.3
Corn flakes	8.5	9.3	.5	78.7	2.6	10.8	1.3	91.3	103.4
Hominy, cooked	79.3	2.2	.2	17.8	.5	2.6	.5	20.6	23.7
Macaroni, cooked	78.4	3.0	1.5	15.8	1.3	3.5	4.0	18.3	25.8
Oatmeal, boiled	84.5	2.8	.5	11.5	.7	3.2	1.3	13.3	17.8
Peas, green, cooked	73.8	6.7	3.4	14.6	1.5	7.8	9.0	16.9	33.7
Rice, boiled	72.5	2.8	.1	24.4	.2	3.2	.3	28.3	31.8

TABLE B—FRUITS

A. Per cent Water	
B. Per cent Protein	
C. Per cent Fat	
D. Per cent Carbohydrate	
E. Per cent Ash	
F. Calories per oz. Protein	
G. Calories per oz. Fat	
H. Calories per oz. Carbohydrate	
I. Calories per oz. Total	

FOOD	A	B	C	D	E	F	G	H	I
Apples	84.6	.4	.5	14.2	.3	.5	1.3	16.5	18.3
Bananas	75.3	1.3	.6	22.0	.8	1.5	1.6	25.6	28.7
Blackberries	86.3	1.3	1.0	10.9	.5	1.5	2.6	12.6	16.7
Dates	15.4	2.1	2.8	78.4	1.3	2.4	7.4	90.9	100.7
Figs	18.8	4.3	.3	74.2	2.4	5.0	.8	86.1	91.9
Grapes	77.4	1.3	1.6	19.2	.5	1.5	4.2	22.3	28.0

	A	B	C	D	E	F	G	H	I
Oranges	86.9	.8	.2	11.6	.5	.9	.5	13.5	14.9
Peaches	89.4	.7	.1	9.4	.4	.8	.3	10.9	12.0
Raisins	14.6	2.6	3.3	76.1	3.4	3.0	8.7	88.3	100.0
Strawberries	90.4	1.0	.6	7.4	.6	1.2	1.6	8.6	11.4

TABLE C—NUTS

A. Per cent Water
B. Per cent Protein
C. Per cent Fat
D. Per cent Carbohydrate
E. Per cent Ash
F. Calories per oz. Protein
G. Calories per oz. Fat
H. Calories per oz. Carbohydrate
I. Calories per oz. Total

FOOD	A	B	C	D	E	F	G	H	I
Almonds	4.8	21.0	54.9	17.4	2.0	24.4	144.9	20.2	189.5
Brazil nuts	5.3	17.0	66.8	7.0	3.9	19.7	176.4	8.1	204.2
Chestnuts	5.9	10.7	7.0	74.2	2.2	12.4	18.5	86.1	117.0
Coconuts	14.1	5.7	50.6	27.9	1.7	6.5	133.6	32.4	172.5
Hickory nuts	3.7	15.4	67.4	11.4	2.1	17.9	177.9	13.2	209.0
Peanuts	9.2	25.8	38.6	24.4	2.0	29.9	101.9	28.3	160.1
Pecans	3.0	11.0	71.2	13.3	1.5	12.8	188.0	15.4	216.2
Pine nuts	6.4	33.9	49.4	6.9	3.4	39.3	130.4	8.0	177.7
Walnuts, black	2.5	27.6	56.3	11.7	1.9	32.0	149.6	13.6	195.2
Walnuts, English	2.5	16.6	63.4	16.1	1.4	19.3	167.4	18.7	205.4

TABLE D—VEGETABLES

A. Per cent Water
B. Per cent Protein
C. Per cent Fat
D. Per cent Carbohydrate
E. Per cent Ash
F. Calories per oz. Protein
G. Calories per oz. Fat
H. Calories per oz. Carbohydrate
I. Calories per oz. Total

FOOD	A	B	C	D	E	F	G	H	I

Asparagus, cooked	91.6	2.1	3.3	2.2	.8	2.4	8.7	2.6	13.7
Beets, cooked	88.6	2.3	.1	7.4	1.6	2.7	.3	8.6	11.6
Cabbage	91.5	1.6	.3	5.6	1.0	1.9	.8	6.5	9.2
Carrots	88.2	1.1	.4	9.3	1.0	1.3	1.1	10.8	13.2
Lettuce	94.7	1.2	.3	2.9	.9	1.4	.8	7.7	9.9
Onions	87.6	1.6	.3	9.9	.6	1.9	.8	11.5	14.2
Potatoes, boiled	75.5	2.5	.1	20.9	1.0	2.9	.3	24.2	27.4
Spinach, cooked	89.8	2.1	4.1	2.6	1.4	2.4	4.8	3.0	10.2
Tomatoes	94.3	.9	.4	3.9	.5	1.0	1.1	4.5	6.6
Turnips	89.6	1.3	.2	8.1	.8	1.5	.5	9.4	11.4

TABLE E—MISCELLANEOUS FOODS

A. Per cent Water

B. Per cent Protein

C. Per cent Fat

D. Per cent Carbohydrate

E. Per cent Ash

F. Calories per oz. Protein

G. Calories per oz. Fat

H. Calories per oz. Carbohydrate

I. Calories per oz. Total

FOOD	A	B	C	D	E	F	G	H	I
Butter	11.0	1.0	85.0		3.0	1.2	224.4		225.6
Cane sugar				100.0				116.0	116.0
Cream	74.0	2.5	18.5	4.5	.5	2.9	48.8	5.2	56.9
Cottage cheese	72.0	20.9	1.0	4.3	1.8	24.2	2.6	5.0	31.8
Eggs	73.7	13.4	10.5		1.0	15.5	27.7		43.2
Honey	18.2	.4		81.2	.2	.5		94.2	94.7
Milk	87.0	3.3	4.0	5.0	.7	3.8	10.6	5.8	20.2
Milk, condensed	68.2	9.6	9.3	11.2	1.7	11.1	24.6	13.0	48.7
Milk, skimmed	90.5	3.4	.3	5.1	.7	3.9	.8	5.9	10.6
Olives, ripe	64.7	1.7	25.0	4.3	3.4	2.0	66.0	5.0	73.0

Thoroughly toasted bread is quite well dextrinized. It is more easily digested, has a sweeter taste than ordinary bread, and in some cases, is more desirable.

Sugar Group

Cane sugar is probably the most important member of the sugar groups. It is obtained from the sugar cane and the sugar beet, the two forms being identical chemically. It can be obtained in a high state of purity, often up to ninety-nine and eight tenths per cent. The English-speaking races use the largest amount of this sugar, in some countries averaging as high as eighty-five pounds per capita a year. Cane sugar is white, crystalline, soluble in water, and has a very sweet taste.

Malt sugar is obtained from grains, such as barley or wheat, by allowing them to sprout. During the sprouting process, there is developed in the grain a ferment that is capable of changing starch to malt sugar. After the malt diastase, as the ferment is called, has had a chance to convert the starch to malt sugar, the sugar is extracted with water, and the resulting solution evaporated to a sirup. This sirup can be evaporated further and the malt sugar or maltose taken out as a solid; but it is usually used in the form of a sirup. This maltose is a natural product to the body, as it is formed by the saliva and the pancreatic juice when they act upon starch.

Milk sugar is found to the extent of about five per cent in cow's milk. It is obtained as a by-product in the manufacture of cheese. The whey, or watery fluid left after the removal of the curd, is evaporated and purified until a fine, white, rather gritty powder, or in some cases a crystalline solid, is obtained. This milk sugar, or lactose, is soluble in water, and has a fairly sweet taste. Lactose is one of the essential food elements for the normal growth of a child or a young animal. Hence one can see why children cannot be reared easily without milk.

Glucose is the most important sugar in the third group of carbohydrates as given above. It is found naturally in many fruits, and is here called grape sugar. It is the normal sugar of human blood, and in this connection, is usually called dextrose. Glucose is made commercially by boiling starch, most frequently cornstarch, in water, to which sulphuric acid has been added up to one to one and one half per cent. After sufficient boiling, the acid is neutralized with lime, and the sugar separated by chemical methods. If the process is carried out carefully, and reasonably pure reagents are used in the process, the result will be a sirup of fair purity and one of value as a food. Impure and poorly made samples of glucose have given this otherwise wholesome sugar a bad name.

Glucose can also be obtained in solid form by continuing the process of purification a few steps beyond the sirup stage. But let it not be forgotten that any of the sugars, taken in large amounts, may overload the digestive system and the liver, and hence they should be used in reasonable amounts.

Levulose, called also fruit sugar, is found in some of the sweet fruits and in bees' honey. The chief sugar of honey is called invert sugar, and is really made up of equal parts of dextrose and levulose. It is present up to seventy-five per cent in good samples of honey. These sugars, properly used, are excellent foods.

Importance of Carbohydrates

The carbohydrates are our chief source of heat and energy, and as previously stated, furnish sixty to sixty-five per cent of the total fuel value of our food. Each ounce of pure carbohydrate yields one hundred sixteen calories of heat when burned. In caloric yield, they are equal to the proteins gram for gram, but yield less than one half that of the fats. If two thousand five hundred calories are again taken as our standard, then sixty per cent would make one thousand five hundred calories to be furnished by the carbohydrates. At one hundred sixteen calories an ounce, we find that it would require thirteen ounces of pure carbohydrate a day to balance this part of our diet.

Other Essential Elements

The inorganic salts or ash of food are just as essential to the body as the other groups of food elements. These essential salts consist of the most common chemical elements, such as soda, potash, lime, magnesia, iron, phosphorus, sulphur, etc. One might expect to find some rare elements in a piece of mechanism as complicated as the human body, but such is not the case. The body salts are of the most common kinds. These salts are found in proper amounts in foods as produced by nature. We cannot take these salts as they are found in the chemical laboratory and use them to good advantage, but we should make sure that we are taking foods that will supply them in the proper amounts. Our best sources of supply are the grains, the fruits, and the vegetables. It is interesting to note that these mineral elements are generally found most abundantly, in the grains at least, in or near the outer coating, and that our high-grade flours are partially robbed of them when the bran and the middlings are removed. The same seems to be true of potatoes. In peeling, a large part of these salts is removed, and thus the real value of this splendid food product is lessened. This is one of the strong arguments for the use of whole wheat flours and other whole grain products. These inorganic salts are needed in the body to keep the various tissues up to their normal in composition. For example, the blood constantly needs some iron to build the red cells. Though the actual amount needed is very small, yet that small amount is exceedingly important to have at hand.

As some of these salts are constantly being eliminated from the body, there must be a constant supply to keep the tissues in equilibrium.

Vitamines

Vitamines are elsewhere considered in this booklet, hence only a very brief summary here. The chemistry of these products is very little understood at present. They were so named by Funk because of their nitrogen content and similarity to ammonia, the name really meaning *vital ammonias*. The term "vital" carries with it the idea of their importance to life. Some persons have questioned this name; but up to the present, it seems to be the best suggested.

The importance of the vitamines in nutrition has been very clearly demonstrated in experiments upon animals, and these experiments have been repeated a sufficient number of times to be conclusive. Animals have been fed upon pure protein, fat, carbohydrate, and salts, but with vitamine removed or destroyed; and although receiving calories enough, they fail to keep up their nutrition. With a simple change of dietary to include a small amount of food containing the vitamine, without any change in the total calories eaten, their nutrition improves quickly, and they come back to a normal state.

Foods rich in vitamine are represented by milk, fresh vegetables, fresh fruits, and whole grain products. Foods poor in these substances are represented by sterilized and preserved milks, dried fruits, dried vegetables, white flour, and polished rice.

Vitamines are reduced or lost by the following processes in the preparation of foods: taking off the coating of grain, overheating, washing out in cooking, and drying.

Importance of Water

Water, although not a food in the sense of yielding fuel value to the body, is a most important agent in all the various chemical processes taking place in the tissues.

Water is the universal solvent; and because of this property, it carries both food and waste to and from the tissues. The average person needs from three to five quarts a day, a part of which is taken as a portion of the food eaten. This leaves from three to five pints to be taken as a drink. Good drinking water should be colorless, odorless, and of an agreeable taste; should be free from organic matter, poisonous metals, and the bacteria of disease; and should be low in nonpoisonous mineral salts—that is, should be reasonably soft.

There are three common classes of water that are used for drinking purposes; namely, rain water, surface water, and ground water. Rain water is the purest if properly collected. Surface water—water from lakes, streams, etc.—is most likely to be contaminated with organic matter and bacteria. Ground water—that is, water from springs and wells—is likely to be the hardest, but is usually free from bacteria of disease unless there is some contamination from the surface. To take a fairly good quantity of water between meals is better than to drink too freely at the meal hour.

Great care should be taken in selecting the supply of drinking water, as when contaminated, it is a very fruitful means for the transmission of diseases, particularly such diseases as typhoid fever. If not certain of the purity of a water supply, one can be sure to destroy all the disease-producing bacteria by boiling the water for a few minutes, then cooling, and drinking as usual.

Simple Dietetic Principles

1. Food should be pleasant to the sight and the taste.

2. Eat slowly. Masticate thoroughly.

3. Do not wash down your food with water or any kind of beverage.

4. Cheerfulness is an important aid to digestion. The mind should be free from care, and the surroundings pleasant.

5. Avoid overeating.

6. There should be between five and six hours' interval between meals, and no food should be taken during this interval.

7. Make your list of foods balance up with about ten per cent protein, twen-

ty-five to thirty per cent fat, and sixty to sixty-five per cent carbohydrate.

8. Eat few kinds of food at a meal, but vary the menu from day to day.

9. Food should be properly cooked to get the best results.

10. Do not eat late at night. The evening meal should be the lightest.

11. Eat green vegetables frequently in season.

12. Fresh fruits are very helpful in the diet.

13. Combine fruits, grains, and nuts.

14. Fruits and coarse vegetables are not a good combination.

15. It is better not to take large quantities of cane sugar and milk together.

16. Do not eat rich and complicated mixtures of food.

17. Flesh meats are expensive, they make the protein high, and are second-hand foods. Their place may easily be supplied by other foods.

18. Avoid excessive amounts of salt.

19. Do not use pepper or other irritating condiments and spices in seasoning your food.

20. Tea and coffee are not foods, and should be entirely dispensed with.

21. Alcohol is a poison, and should be entirely eliminated from the menu.

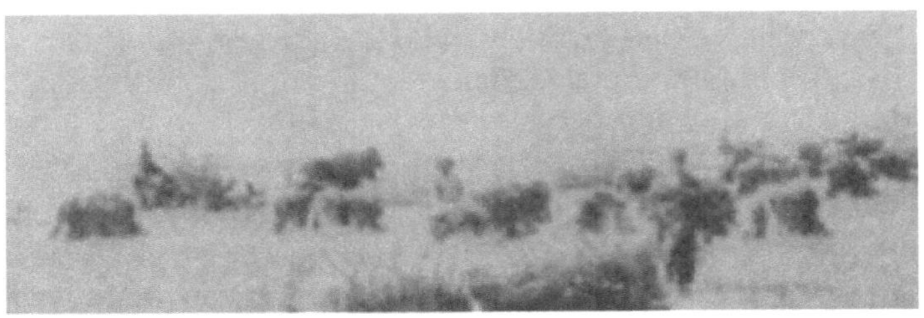

NECESSARY KNOWLEDGE TO CAREFUL PLANNING

TO thousands of home-keepers the requirements are new: a correct knowledge of proteids, of carbohydrates, of calories is unfamiliar to them. They cannot grasp what is asked of them, in a day or a week or a month. Suddenly has housekeeping been transformed from a daily round to a science and a business.... It all calls for intelligent study and the most careful planning. It is not a small "bit," it is a full-sized job: never has the American woman faced a bigger job. As she does it or fails of doing it, will this great country win or lose the war.—*Ladies' Home Journal.*

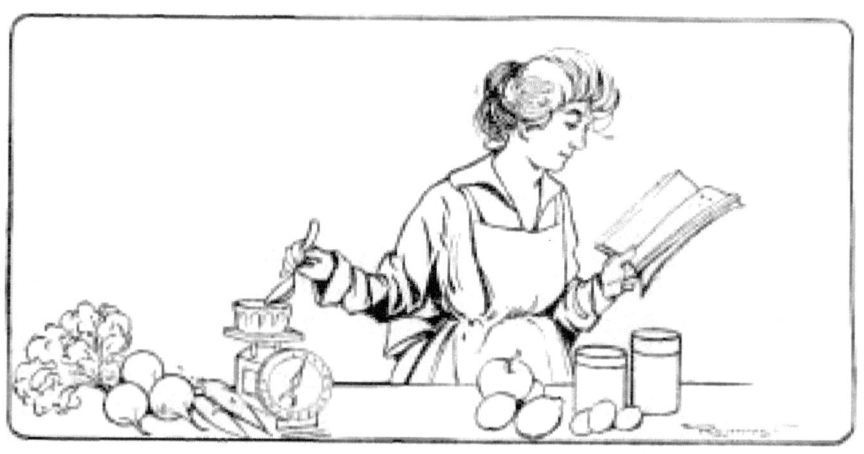

VITAMINES AND CALORIES

BY
D. D. COMSTOCK, M.D.

*for years Medical Superintendent of Glendale
Sanitarium, Glendale, California*

The body is a machine, intricate, complicated, "fearfully and wonderfully" constructed. In one way, it is simple in its operations; but in another, so ultrascientific in the detail of its automatic control, and so deep in the mysteries of its chemical processes, that the investigation of ages has not been able to fathom its greater scientific depths, and bring to the surface a knowledge of its ultimate structure and its wonderful workings. The Master Designer of the living machine so adjusted its mechanism that in its original environment and relationship, its care would be easy, and the laws of its preservation few and exceedingly simple.

Like most machines, the human machine requires the impartation of energy. Similarly, also, this is supplied by the combustion of certain carbonaceous substances. It needs constant repair. These and its other needs are all furnished in the daily food supply.

The life of this machine can be greatly lengthened by intelligent care, or shortened by neglect and abuse. Its efficiency may be similarly affected. While one cannot hear the pounding of the engine or the rattling of the machinery, yet the machine is damaged if run under too high a pressure and at too great speed.

There are seven classes of the essential elemental food substances,—proteins, fats, carbohydrates, vitamines, salts, cellulose, and water. The ideal diet is one in which these seven elements are regularly supplied to the body in the amounts required to meet its daily needs. A person living close to nature, receiving his food first-handed, direct from nature's health food factory, and eating it with only the cooking and seasoning necessary, and with a reasonable variety, would probably find his diet sufficient, and the elements in about the proper proportions; and with an honest appetite, steadied by a little temperate-in-all-things ballast, he probably would not go far astray as to the proper amounts. But unfortunately, the average individual is not living close to nature. Much that is artificial has come in. Our appetites are capricious, deceitful, and unreasonable. Our foods come to us processed, cartonned, and tinned, often embalmed, devitalized, or adulterated. They are often served to us so disguised that we cannot tell whether their nutritive substance has been concentrated or diluted, or indeed whether or not the body will recognize it as having any nutritive value at all, despite its pleasing flavor. Therefore, in order that the ideal may be approximated to a reasonable and practical degree, we must have some knowledge not only of the needs of the body, but also of these food elements, and how their values may be estimated in the various food substances.

The foods that enter into the make-up of the body and supply its heat and energy are three,—protein, fat, and carbohydrate. While the salts to a certain extent enter into the body structure, they have but little to do with heat and energy production. The remaining food classes are adjuncts, their use being simply to make possible the utilization, by the body, of the tissue and fuel foods. The cellulose assists mechanically in digestion; the water furnishes the necessary fluid; and the vitamines provide the battery, as it were, which sets the whole apparatus in motion.

The Heat Unit

Of the many persons who, for economical or hygienic reasons, have tried to adjust their diet better, some have undertaken the task without a fundamental knowledge of the physiological and caloric value of foods, their composition, or the nutritional needs of the body, and have done themselves more harm than good. It is possible for us to measure the value of our foods, and to express it in terms of heat units; and with a knowledge of the bodily needs, we may supply ourselves with foods in approximately the amounts needed, and in the best combinations. Food oxidized in the body produces the same amount of heat as that burned outside the body, and the instrument by which the heat value of any substance is determined is called a calorimeter. The unit of measure of heat is called the calorie or heat unit.

The calorimeter consists of a double chamber, the outer one containing a given quantity of water. The inner chamber is thus surrounded by a water jacket. In it is placed a definite amount of pure, water-free food to be tested; for example, an ounce of sugar. By means of an electric connection, the sugar is ignited and burned, and the heat produced thereby is imparted to the water in the outer chamber. When the process is complete, the difference in the temperature of the water is noted, and the amount of heat generated is computed. The calorie is the amount of heat necessary to raise the temperature of one pound of water four degrees F., or one kilogram one degree C. In this way, the heat values of pure protein, fat, starch, and sugar have been determined. In the laboratories of the United States government, the composition and caloric value of practically every food substance known has been worked out. Any person can have access to these tables of food values by applying to the government, or by purchasing from almost any bookstore any one of the several books on food values, that are on the market. (See pages 23-27 of this book.)

The heat value of a gram of pure, water-free protein—for example, the casein of milk, egg albumen, or fiber of meat—is a trifle more than four calories. That of pure starch or sugar is also four calories. Fat is more than double this value, one gram yielding nine and three tenths calories. Since an ounce equals about thirty grams, the number of calories to an ounce is determined by multiplying the above figures by thirty. Different kinds of food vary greatly in the proportion of the food elements and also of the water and cellulose they contain. (Cellulose has no fuel value in the human body.) We therefore find a great variation as to their caloric values also. For example, one heaping tablespoonful of home-baked beans will weigh about fifty grams, thirty of which is water and cellulose. Its total caloric value is one hundred, divided among protein fifteen, fat forty (the fat has largely been added), and carbohydrate forty-five. Contrast with this the same quantity of mashed turnips. One heaping tablespoonful will weigh about seventy grams, of which sixty-five is water and cellulose. Its total fuel value is three calories.

By a little study, one may very readily become familiar with the approximate values of the more common foods, and be able to arrive at some conclusion in regard to the correctness of one's daily food ration as to amount and proportions. Many would be surprised to see how far short their diet comes of the ideal.

It is easy to remember that an ordinary slice of bread—about three and one half inches square—contains approximately one hundred calories; an average egg, sixty-five; a glass of milk, one hundred fifty; an average potato, one hundred twenty-five; a tablespoonful of gravity cream, fifty; the usual serving of cooked cereal, seventy-five to one hundred; vegetables, except potatoes, an ordinary serving, twenty-five to fifty, depending on the amount of fat or milk added as seasoning; legumes, average serving, one hundred to one hundred fifty. Desserts are usually high in value, ranging from one hundred twenty-five calories in the usual serving of simple custard or junket to three hundred fifty or more in the usual one sixth of some pies, or the ordinary piece of cake.

Housewives who wish to go into the question of foods thoroughly, and combine the science with the art of cookery, may arrange a table of the staples and raw food that ordinarily enter into their various recipes, somewhat after the following, the items of which have been taken at random from such a list or table already prepared and in use:

| A. *Food* |
| B. *Measure* |
| C. *Weight* |
| D. *Protein* |

A	B	C	D	E	F	G
E. *Fat*						
F. *Carbohydrate*						
G. *Total*						
Flour	1 cup	5 oz.	80	25	419	524
Eggs, average	each	1½ oz.	23	40	0	63
Milk, whole	1 cup	8 oz.	30	88	46	164
Sugar, granulated	1 cup	7½ oz.	0	0	840	840
Butter	1 cup	8 oz.	0	1,744	0	1,744
Butter	1 tablespoon	½ oz.	0	109	0	109

If the housewife desires to know the food value of a cake, for instance, that she is about to bake, whose recipe calls for two cups flour, one and one half cups sugar, one half cup butter, four eggs, she can very easily find out by consulting her table; as:

		A	B	C	D
A. *Protein*					
B. *Fat*					
C. *Carbohydrate*					
D. *Total*					
2 cups flour	=	160	50	838	1,048
1½ cups sugar	=	0	0	1,260	1,260
½ cup butter	=	0	872	0	872
4 eggs	=	92	160	0	252
Totals		252	1,082	2,098	3,432

If the cake is cut into twelve servings, the value of each may be determined by dividing each of these sums by twelve. Thus each piece will represent in value, protein, twenty-one calories; fat, ninety calories; carbohydrate, one hundred seventy-five calories; total, two hundred eighty-six calories.

The number of calories needed by the individual varies with height, age, sex, climate, and state of muscular activity; but for the average person, two thousand calories daily may be taken as a working basis. If one is engaged in active muscular labor, the requirement may be three thousand or more. Many persons of sedentary habits do better on less than two thousand. Other things being equal, men need about ten per cent more than women. Children need about ten per cent more than adults. An obese individual, or one suffering from the results of imperfect oxidation, as manifested in rheumatism, neuralgia, and myalgia, may do well for a time on as low an allowance as one thousand one hundred to one thousand two hundred food units daily, experiencing marked relief from symptoms, and if obese, a reduction in weight of from one to four pounds a week.

It should be kept in mind that the amount of protein needed is quite constant, and does not vary with one's state of activity, as does the demand for the fats and the carbohydrates. From two hundred to two hundred fifty calories of this element are needed daily, even though the total ration be low. If one does well on the low ration suggested above, the protein should not be lowered proportionately, as would be the tendency. This is the repair substance, which the body, not being able to store up, must have supplied to it in regular daily amounts.

Excess in eating is often due to the use of certain concentrated foods. A teaspoonful of olive oil contains forty calories; the ordinary pat of butter (one fourth ounce), fifty calories; a heaping teaspoonful of sugar, forty calories; one English walnut, thirty-three calories; a fair sized olive, twenty calories. While these are good foods, they should be eaten with due regard for their high energy value, that the proper food balance be not disturbed. After eating a good square meal, the average individual calls for the dessert, which, with its accompaniments, actually constitutes a second meal; as, for example, a serving of pie, three hundred fifty calories; its cheese accompaniment, another one hundred calories; a few stuffed dates, another one hundred calories; a few nuts and raisins and a cup of chocolate bringing the total value of this second meal forced upon the body up to seven hundred or eight hundred calories.

Vegetables of themselves are low in caloric value, their importance being due to the cellulose, salts, and vitamines they contain. But they are usually prepared with so much butter or cream that as served they have a high caloric value in fat. Lean meat is practically pure protein, and the tendency of the meat eater is to get an excess of this element. The vegetarian often goes to the other extreme, his diet showing a deficiency in protein, with an excess of fats and carbohydrates. That the protein balance be kept normal is an important matter, for a person may at one and the same time be suffering from the results of a deficient diet and also from the effects of overeating. The protein needed daily is from ten to thirteen per cent of the total ration. If the total daily ration is but one thousand five hundred calories, the protein should still be two hundred calories, and therefore thirteen per cent of the total. Thus if a person is living on foods containing less than ten per cent, there is danger of not getting enough of this important element. Much of the food eaten is less than ten per cent protein, because of the addition to it of fat and sugar in large amounts.

So-called meat substitutes should be high in the percentage of protein, in order to make up for the butter, sugar, oils, olives, desserts, fruits, and other very low protein foods that enter so largely into one's dietary. The question has been asked, Why object to the addition of fat to a meat substitute, since it does not actually reduce the quantity of protein, though it does relatively? In reply, it may be said that the relative reduction makes necessary an excess of the nonnitrogenous foods, to get enough protein; and even though one's capacity should receive it comfortably, still the objection to the excess aliment remains.

A study of food composition and values will enable the housewife so to plan her meals that the various elements may be served to her family in the proper proportions. A knowledge of calories, and an intelligent application of the principles involved in these questions of nutrition, will enable any housewife to reduce the cost of feeding her family from twenty-five to fifty per cent, which would be worth while from an economical standpoint, not to mention the advantage to be realized healthwise.

Vitamines

Says Lusk, "It has thus far been shown that nutrition means fuel for the machinery, new parts with which to repair the machine, and minute quantities of vitamines, which produce a harmonious interaction between the materials in the food and their host."

In the words of another investigator, "The study of dietetics from the standpoint of the vitamines has only just begun." Sufficient has been learned and demonstrated about them, however, to show that they play a most important part in nutrition and in vital tissue processes. Since they are so little understood, a complete definition is not yet possible. The pure vitamine, it seems, cannot be isolated, so their exact chemical nature is not known. The chemical process necessary to free it is no sooner begun than the vitamine is apparently decomposed, and all trace of it is lost. One is reminded of the efforts of some early investigators to submit living protoplasm to a chemical analysis, they hoping thereby to reveal the mysteries of physical life itself; but at the first intrusion, this subtle something flees, taking its secrets with it, and leaving us only the empty shell of dead protein matter. While the activities and manifestations of life are seen on every hand in animal and plant, we are but little the wiser as to what life really is.

Vitamines seem to stand closely related to the living process in the tissue cells. Some investigators have thought them to be the mother substances of the various bodily ferments and internal secretions, any disturbance of which produces serious constitutional troubles. Therefore the continuous use of a diet lacking in any of these mother substances would of necessity lead to a deficiency of these absolutely essential vital secretions and ferments.

Vitamines and Disease

Years were spent in investigation before it was found out that beriberi, a disease of the Orient, could be cured and prevented by the addition, to the diet, of certain nutritive elements in the covering of the rice, that are ordinarily removed in the polishing process, and thrown away. Just what these nutritive elements were, was not understood; but the fact remained that a diet of polished rice resulted in symptoms of beriberi, while a diet of the unpolished grain was sufficient to prevent any manifestations of the disease. In Java, where the people lived largely on whole rice, beriberi was unknown. For years, the fact had been recognized, that sailors living on canned and preserved foods sooner or later developed scurvy, which could be quickly cured by an addition of fresh vegetables or the juice of fruits, especially lemons and oranges, to the diet. In 1535, when all but three of Cartier's one hundred ten sailors had scurvy, he cured them all by giving them a decoction of fresh pine needles. Babies fed on Pasteurized milk often develop infantile scurvy.

Convincing Experiments

Vitamines are made only in nature's laboratory. The body cannot make them, therefore mother's milk is deficient in vitamine if her diet is. This is demonstrated in a decided way in the Philippine Islands, where the diet is deficient in the vitamine preventing beriberi. Among the Filipinos, one half the deaths take place before the end of the first year of age; and in these infants, one half the deaths are due to beriberi. Pellagra, a disease of obscure ætiology, or cause, manifests itself principally among a class of people who live on a monotonous diet of corn bread, bacon, soda biscuit, and sirup. Some authorities are quite convinced that it is a "deficiency" disease. Also rickets, eczema, pyorrhea, and a number of other diseases of obscure cause are beginning to be regarded as being, in part at least, deficiency diseases. A predisposition to tuberculosis and other infections may be of similar cause. There are probably a number, possibly many, of these vitamine substances. At least two have been quite fully demonstrated, — the one preventing scurvy, and the one preventing beriberi.

The experiments of Cosimir Funk, a Russian, are convincing. He was able to produce experimental beriberi in pigeons by feeding them for three weeks on polished rice, then readily to cure them of the disease by feeding the polishings from the same rice, showing that in the rice polishings are certain elements absolutely essential to life. He finally isolated what appeared to be this substance, one pound of the polishings yielding about three grains of the material. Injecting under the skin of pigeons dying of beriberi one third of a grain of this crystalline substance, he was able not only to make them perfectly well in a few hours, but to keep them in health for three weeks with but the one dose, even though they were continued on a diet of polished rice. Funk named this wonderful life-giving substance vitamine, because its effects were life-giving, and chemically it seemed to belong to the amines.

Where Found

Vitamines are found in plants, and especially in their seeds. Fresh meat and raw milk contain them, although animals seem incapable of making them. In summer, milk is richer in them than in winter, because of the difference in feed for the cattle. They are contained also in yolks of eggs, whole grains, potatoes, carrots, beans, peas, lentils—in fact, practically all green garden vegetables, and fruit. In the grains, they are found in the dark layer near the outer surface or branny layer, and in the germ. In potatoes and other vegetables, they lie immediately under the skin. Yeast bread contains more than baking powder breads.

Vitamines are lost by the processing of grains; that is, by the removal of the outer layers, which contain most of these substances. Hence the whole grain should be included in the flour. They are also destroyed by the subjection of foods to too high a temperature. It is therefore best to cook cereals at a low temperature, as in a fireless cooker. The vitamines are sacrificed in the drying of foods, and in the paring of vegetables. If potatoes are boiled, there is great advantage in boiling them in their "jackets," in which case the vitamines and the salts are not lost. If they are pared before they are boiled, the potato water should not be thrown away, as it is rich in vitamines, salts, and protein. Parboiling of other vegetables is objectionable for the same reason. Soda and baking powder and similar chemicals seem to destroy the vitamines. This is one reason why yeast breads are better than baking powder breads. Furthermore, in yeast fermentation, the vitamine preventing beriberi is actually formed, but not the vitamine preventing scurvy. The natural foods that require cooking to make them edible and wholesome contain vitamines which are not destroyed thereby if the cooking is done in the most wholesome and hygienic way.

A WORD OF ADVICE TO WOMEN

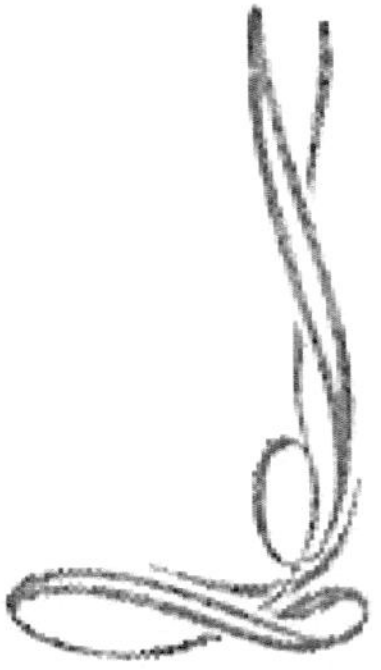

STAY at home and work. Do not rush into some romantic and picturesque bit of action to the detriment of your home duties. Work in your homes, and do whatever you can outside; the humbler and more inconspicuous your accomplishment is, the more it may be needed. There are enough women who will snatch at what is accompanied by the limelight. Make your contribution of personal service without thought of self, and keep on to the end. — *Lord Northcliffe.*

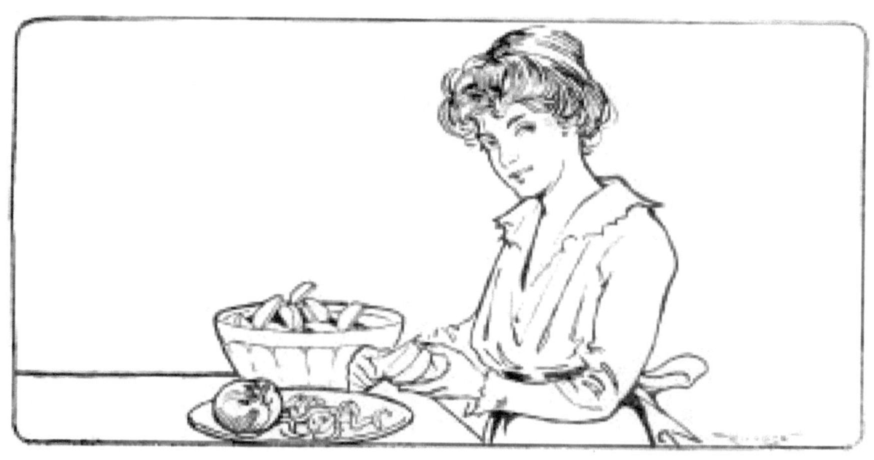

FRUITS AND THEIR DIETETIC VALUE
BY
GEORGE A. THOMASON, M.D., L.R.C.S., L.R.C.P.

No other class of foods more delightfully or deliciously contribute to the needs of the body than fruit. Fresh from the lap of Nature, lavishly supplied, and delightful to the eye, fruit makes most satisfying appeal to the appetite of every one, from the quite indifferent to the most discriminating epicure. Most easy of digestion, in fact, practically predigested, fruit is most appropriate for all people both in sickness and in health, and at all periods of life, from babyhood to extreme age.

Fruit is made up of water, sugar, acids, some proteid, and organic salts. Water is by far the largest constituent of fruit, being seventy-five to eighty-five per cent. The water of fruit is of the greatest possible purity, being doubly distilled, first as rain, then as sap, drawn and filtered through the tree.

The sugar of fruit is one of the most easily digested forms, that of levulose. The starch of the unripe fruit is converted into sugar in the ripening process, or in the cooking of partially ripened fruit. Sugar is present in varying amounts in fruits, averaging from five to ten per cent. A well ripened banana contains twenty-one per cent of sugar, dates about fifty per cent, while grapes contain from fourteen to twenty per cent.

The outward appearance of the fruit is often a fairly reliable indication of the amount of sugar. Trielle has observed that fruits with yellow skins contain much sugar, and have a very penetrating odor. Fruits with red skins contain a medium amount of sugar, and have a pleasant, delicate perfume. Fruits with a reddish brown skin usually contain much sugar, and have very little perfume.

As showing its perfectly digested state, demonstrations have proved that fruit sugar may be injected directly into the blood, from which it will be utilized in nourishing the body. This is in marked contrast with ordinary cane sugar, which, if injected directly into the blood, is expelled through the kidneys, the body being unable to appropriate it as such from the blood.

Fruit sugar may be eaten in practically unlimited quantities. It supplies the body with heat and energy in the most available form. For this reason, fruit when eaten will quickly relieve the sense of exhaustion.

Fruit Acids

The acids of fruits give to them their delightful and appetizing flavors. Fruits in the unripe state contain tannic acid, a marked astringent. The gastric and peristaltic woes of the small boy the night following the green apple episode are due to the tannic acid the unripe fruit contains. The three chief acids of fruit are citric acid, found in oranges, lemons, and grapefruit; malic acid, as found in apples, pears, peaches, and similar fruits; and tartaric acid, as found in grapes. These are organic acids, recognized and readily digested by the body.

The acids of fruits are remarkable peptogens; that is, they stimulate the appetite and promote the flow of the digestive juices. Fruit acids are most efficient disinfectants. Some years ago, an eminent medical authority of this country, in a representative medical gathering, said, "We are as yet without a satisfactory medicinal intestinal disinfectant." In fruit acids, we possess such an agent in a most desirable form. No germ, disease-producing or otherwise, can live in the presence of fruit acid. Fruit acids can be taken practically *ad libitum*. Fruit acids taken freely by mouth or diluted and injected into the bowel, most efficiently asepticize the intestinal canal. Three or four pints of water to which the juice of one lemon has been added, injected into the bowel following a cleansing enema, will thoroughly destroy disease-producing bacteria in the colon. Flushing the bowel frequently with such a solution is one of the most efficient known means of successfully combating the fetid summer diarrheas of children.

The proteid or nitrogenous element of fruits, as well as their fatty element, may be passed over with little consideration. Fruit contains little proteid; and aside from the olive, there is almost no fat in fruit. The fat of the ripe olive, however, is one of the most delicious and digestible forms of fat. Ripe olives contain about fifty per cent fat. Olive oil can be mixed with water; therefore it readily mixes with the intestinal juices, and is most easily digested.

Fruit Salts

The salts of fruit are most desirable, being so essential in tissue building. Some of the most important of these salts are potash, lime, phosphoric acid, and iron. Deficiency of the lime salts in the bones of children produces conditions of bone softening, or rickets. This can be largely prevented by adding fruit to the diet of these afflicted children, using especially grapes, oranges, lemons, and grapefruit, which contain high percentages of lime salts.

The condition of anæmia is a lack of iron in the blood. This cannot be replaced by medicinal or metallic iron, as the body is unable to appropriate these inorganic substances; but the iron in fruit is perfectly adapted to the body needs. Plums, cherries, and especially strawberries and currants contain considerable iron, and are most helpful in the treatment of anæmic conditions.

It is perfectly apparent that fruits possess qualities and constituents that make them of the greatest value as an essential part of the daily ration to nourish and energize the body, and to promote vital activities in the maintenance of strength and healthful vigor. Fruit is also an exceedingly important and efficient factor in restoring to normal function tissues and organs that have become vitiated and are functionating abnormally.

In spite of the widespread opinion to the contrary, it can be positively asserted that fruit is of great service in the prevention as well as in the treatment of rheumatism and gout. The prejudice against the use of fruit in rheumatism originated with the idea that the acids of fruit tend to acidify the body. Quite the reverse is true. The acids of fruit, when taken into the body, are promptly converted into the alkali carbonates, thus increasing the alkalinity of the blood, tending greatly to benefit and cure the rheumatic condition, as well as to lessen the general tendency to the formation of various calculi, or stones, in the kidneys, the urinary bladder, and the gall bladder.

Fruit and Obesity

A fruit diet is of great value in obesity. An exclusive fruit diet may be taken to the greatest possible advantage by the too corpulent who wish to reduce in weight. For this purpose, fruit has the advantage of satisfying the appetite while at the same time contributing very little nutrition to the body. The free use of fruit is the method par excellence for overcoming constipation. The eating of a half dozen raw prunes before breakfast, or the taking of the juice of one or two oranges, will in the majority of cases be all that is necessary to maintain regular bowel activity.

For an overworked liver, the so-called "bilious" state, fruit is the best of all means of relief. Auto-intoxication due to an excess of poisons circulating in the blood, is treated most naturally and efficiently by a fruit diet.

The natural diuretic properties of fruit are very well known. Nearly all fruits stimulate the kidneys to greater activity, but watermelon is of particular service in this respect.

Fruit and fruit juices greatly aid in successfully combating alcoholism. The acid of the fruit juices help materially in quenching the abnormal thirst.

There are but few individuals who would not be benefited by an occasional exclusive fruit meal; and in many cases, this can be maintained with greatest benefit for even several days. This is a very popular method of treatment in Europe, particularly in Switzerland, where the "grape cure" is utilized. Patients are placed upon a diet of grapes alone for several weeks, consuming from seven to ten pounds of grapes a day. Wonderful results are recorded at these resorts in the treatment of rheumatism, gout, obesity, constipation, intestinal catarrh, liver and kidney disorders, high blood pressure, arterial sclerosis, or hardening of the arteries, and many more physical disabilities.

Certain fruits, especially tart apples, are of great value in the treatment of diabetes, lessening the toxæmia of this condition, as well as mitigating the abnormal thirst that is so frequent and often distressing an accompaniment of this condition.

In the eating of fruit, some care must be exercised not to swallow large seeds or fruit pits. While the danger of appendicitis from fruit seeds' becoming lodged in the appendix has been greatly exaggerated, yet fruit seeds have occasionally been found in the appendix, and proved the exciting cause of the inflammation which followed. Cases are on record of children who have swallowed considerable quantities of grape seeds, suffering for months of colic, and being only relieved by discharging quantities of these seeds during energetic purgation.

It has been said that fruit is "gold in the morning, silver at noon, and lead at night." But fruit is golden all the time. This wonderful gift, one of the greatest and best physical gifts of an all-wise Providence, cannot be prized to highly; for it is considered sufficiently valuable to endure for both time and eternity. Of the first man and woman, it was said that they might eat of the fruit of the trees of the garden; and it is said of the inhabitants of the renewed earth, during eternity, that "they shall plant vineyards, and eat the fruit of them."

TOO much good food makes one auto-toxic. Too muck fun makes one asinine. But keep sunny. A cheerful disposition, a happy temperament, is the master key that unlocks more secrets, more riches, more success, than anything else. A sunny temper is an "aroma whose fragrance fills the air with an odor of Paradise." Bury everything that makes you unhappy and discordant, everything that cramps your freedom and worries you. Bury it before it buries you. Adopt the sundial's motto, "I record none but hours of sunshine." — *Thomason.*

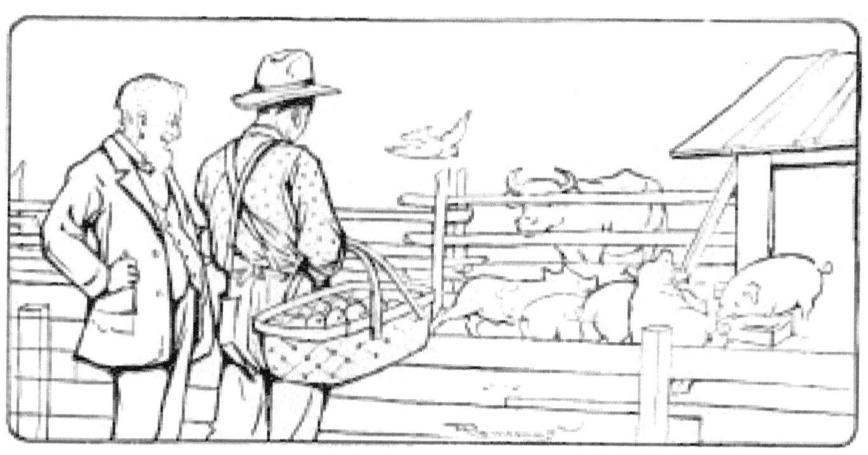

TEN REASONS FOR A FLESHLESS DIET

BY

A. W. TRUMAN, A.B., M.D.

*Superintendent of Loma Linda Sanitarium, Loma
Linda, California; Professor of Neurology, Loma
Linda College*

1. The Strength Delusion

Every movement we make, every thought we think, and every heart throb, involves waste and the expenditure of energy. There is a constant breaking down of our tissues; and the food ingested is the source of the material for repair. By its oxidation, digestion, and assimilation, energy is liberated for life's varied activities.

The primary object of taking food is, in the words of the wise man, "for strength, and not for drunkenness." Any one who makes the pleasure of eating the chief requisite will some day find, by a disordered stomach and a clogged liver, that eating has ceased to be a pleasure.

The idea has long been current that superior qualities of body and mind come from eating flesh food; but the verdict of science, after long observation and careful investigation and various experiments, is rapidly reversing this opinion.

The experiments of Prof. Russell H. Chittenden, president of the American Physiological Society, and director of the Sheffield Scientific School at Yale, are convincing. His elaborate investigations, extending over long periods of time, prove that persons of widely varying habits of life, temperament, occupation, and constitution, can maintain and even heighten their mental and physical vigor while subsisting upon a diet containing but one half the usual amount of protein, and in which the flesh is reduced to a minimum or is entirely absent.

The subjects of the first experiment were three physicians, three professors, and a clerk,—men of sedentary and chiefly of mental occupation. For a period of six months, they were required to reduce the amount of meat and other protein food about one half. "Their weight remained stationary; but they improved in general health, and experienced a quite remarkable increase of mental clearness and energy."

Chittenden's Researches

For his next experiment, Professor Chittenden used a detachment of twenty soldiers from the hospital corps of the United States army, "representing a great variety of types of different ages, nationality, temperament, and degrees of intelligence." For a period of six months, these men lived upon a ration in which the proteid was reduced to one third the usual amount, and the flesh to five sixths of an ounce daily. There was a slight gain in weight, "the general health was well maintained, and with suggestions of improvement that are frequently so marked as to challenge attention." "Most conspicuous, however," remarks Professor Chittenden, "was the effect observed on the muscular strength of the various subjects.... Without exception, we note a phenomenal gain in strength which demands explanation." There was an average gain in strength for each subject of about fifty per cent.

For the third experiment, Professor Chittenden secured as subjects a group of eight leading athletes of Yale, all in training trim. For five months, they subsisted upon a diet comprising from one half to one third the quantity of protein food they had been in the habit of eating. "Gymnasium tests showed in every man a truly remarkable gain in strength and endurance."

Fisher's Experiments

Dr. Irving Fisher, professor of political economy of Yale University, concluded a series of experiments testing the endurance of forty-nine persons, about thirty of the number being flesh abstainers. The first endurance test was that of "holding the arms horizontally." The flesh eaters averaged ten minutes. The flesh abstainers averaged forty-nine minutes. The longest time for a flesh eater was twenty-two minutes. The maximum time for a flesh abstainer was two hundred minutes. The second endurance test was that of "deep knee bending." The flesh eaters averaged three hundred eighty-three times, the flesh abstainers eight hundred thirty-three times. Professor Fisher explains the results on the basis that "flesh foods contain in themselves fatigue poisons of various kinds, which naturally aggravate the action of the fatigue poisons produced in the body."

Dr. J. Ioteyko, head of the laboratory at the University of Brussels, compared the endurance of seventeen vegetarians with that of twenty-five carnivores, students of the University of Brussels. "Comparing the two sets of subjects on the basis of mechanical work, it is found that the vegetarians surpassed the carnivores on the average by fifty-three per cent."

Professor Fisher remarks, "These investigations, with those of Combe of Lausanne, Metchnikoff, and Tisier of Paris, as well as Herter and others in the United States, seem gradually to be demonstrating that the fancied strength from meat is like the fancied strength from alcohol, an illusion."

Tests in Germany

Professor Rubner, of Berlin, "one of the world's foremost students of hygiene," read a paper before the recent International Congress of Hygiene and Demography on the "Nutrition of the People," in which he said: "It is a fact that the diet of the well-to-do is not in itself physiologically justified; it is not even healthful; for on account of the false notions of the strengthening effect of meat, too much meat is used by young and old, and this is harmful."

In the long distance races in Germany, the flesh abstainers have invariably been easy victors. Upon this point, Professor Von Norden, in his monumental work on "Metabolism and Practical Medicine," says: "In Germany at least, in these competitive races, the vegetarian is ahead of the meat eater. The non-vegetarian cannot compete with the vegetarian in the matter of endurance in these long distance walks. The vegetarian is ahead in the matter of rapid pedestrian feats."

A few years ago, a well-known athlete, Dr. Deighton, walked from the southernmost point of England to the northernmost point of Scotland, a distance of almost a thousand miles, in twenty-four days and four hours. His chief subsistence en route was a much advertised meat juice. Mr. George Allen, who for a number of years had subsisted upon a strict non-flesh diet, undertook the same task, which he accomplished in a little less than seventeen days, that is, in seven days less time.

As in the heat engine, energy for light, heat, or power does not come from burning copper, lead, or iron filings, but from carbonaceous materials, as coal, coke, fuel oils, etc., so in the human body, energy for warmth and muscular effort comes not from oxidizing the metal repair foods, the proteins, but from those foods which are rich in carbon, the starches and the sugars, called the carbohydrates.

2. Flesh Food a Stimulant

Whence then come these "illusions," these "false notions of the strengthening effect of meat"? They come from the fact that foods of this class are stimulating. A stimulant is a counterfeit for strength. It is a physical deceiver. It makes a person believe he is strong because he "feels" strong, when it is not true at all. That which is interpreted as strength is only nervous excitement. A stimulant never builds up; it only stirs up. While pretending to contribute energy, it actually robs the body of strength. The resort to stimulants to whip up the flagging energies of the body is an effort to trick nature in playing the game of life. It is like borrowing money. Some day the principal must be returned with interest to a relentless creditor.

Beef tea contains less than one per cent nourishment, but one can get the same kind of exhilaration from a cup of beef tea as from a cup of brandy. This is due to the drug effect of the beef tea, which is a solution of the waste products, the poisonous extractives, of the meat. Every animal organism is constantly throwing off these extractives, such as urea, uric acid, creatinine, etc. The kidneys have no other function than the removal of poisons. If an animal is deprived of the use of its kidneys, it will die of self-poisoning in a few days. When an animal is slaughtered and the blood ceases to circulate, this stream of urinary products on its way to the kidneys for excretion stops in the tissues, and is devoured by the consumer with the flesh.

Friedenwald and Ruhrah, in their book "Diet in Health and Disease," say: "The extractives are probably of no value either as a source of energy or in the formation of tissues. They act as stimulants and appetizers, and it has been stated that the craving some individuals have for meat is in reality a desire for the extractives."

Armand Gautier, the eminent French dietitian, says on this point, "Like the opium smoker, the individual who accustoms himself to meat, feels that he misses it when he does not take the usual excess."

If the poisonous waste products be removed from meat, it is insipid, and is no more stimulating than the same amount of bread.

3. *Ptomaine Poisoning*

The seeds of death and decay are in every animal organism; and just as soon as the heart ceases to throb, and the arteries cease to pulsate, and the spark of life leaves the animal, decomposition begins. These putrefactive changes often result in the formation of violent poisons, called ptomaines. The word "ptomaine" comes from a Greek word meaning *carcass*, or *cadaver*; and the poisons are variously called putrefactive alkaloid, animal alkaloid, etc. The presence of fatal amounts of these poisons in flesh may not be betrayed by any change in appearance, odor, or taste. The common practice of keeping meat until it becomes tender, or "ripens," is simply waiting for decomposition to advance until the meat fiber is softened by the process of decay. Canned meats are especially liable to contain the poisonous ptomaine.

4. *Unbalances the Diet*

It is of primary importance that one should guard against consuming excessive quantities of any kind of food material, but there is a difference. Should we take an excess of starches or sugars, provision has been made for storing a certain amount in the form of fat, or as glycogen in the liver and the muscles; but no provision is found for storing an excess of protein. An excess of this food element is of particular injury to the body. The extensive experiments of Professors Chittenden, Fisher, and other scientific workers, have shown that for efficient nutrition, we require that only one tenth of the daily intake of food should be of the structure-building, tissue-repairing protein. In the laboratory of nature, the food elements have been so combined by the plants, that the protein element is very low; and thus a diet selected from the natural products of the earth is not only free from uric acid and other waste products, but is already balanced. The addition of flesh food—which does not contain any starch—to the menu, at once raises the protein constituent too high.

5. *Bright's Disease and High Blood Pressure*

The waste products in the blood arising from excess of protein are a leading cause of Bright's disease, auto-intoxication, arteriosclerosis, and high blood pressure. These maladies are often associated in the same individual, and frequently have a common origin. Sir William Osler, in his "Principle and Practice of Medicine," writes: "I am more and more impressed with the part played by overeating in inducing arteriosclerosis." "There are many cases in which there is no other factor." Dr. Alexander Haig, of London, states that uric acid makes the blood "collaemic" or viscous, and then the heart has difficulty to pump it through the capillaries. Hence the blood pressure increases. Isaac Ott, in his textbook on physiology, says on this point, "Burton-Opitz has shown that hunger reduces viscosity, and meat diet raises it to a great height, whilst carbohydrates and fat diet give average values to it."

In the colon, flesh foods rapidly undergo decomposition, giving rise to numerous poisons, which are absorbed into the blood, and are toxic to the nervous system, and cast an additional burden upon the liver and the kidneys. These are a sort of dietetic clinkers, which throw nature's delicate machinery out of adjustment, and produce various symptoms of auto-intoxication. Bouchard found that the fecal and urinary excrement of carnivorous animals is twice as poisonous when injected into rabbits as that from a herbivorous animal. The former also emits a strong odor, and the fecal discharges are offensively repulsive. Dr. Haig, before quoted, also asserts that "Bright's disease is the result of our meat-eating and tea-drinking habits; and as these habits are common, so also is the disease."

6. *Tuberculosis, Ulcer, Cancer, and Appendicitis*

While it is true that tuberculosis is more frequently contracted through the use of tuberculous milk than from tuberculous meat, the latter source of infection cannot be ignored. Numerous cases of tuberculosis have been reported where the infection could be directly traced to the flesh of tuberculous animals.

Dr. E. C. Shroeder, of the Bureau of Animal Industry of the United States Department of Agriculture, says: "That ten per cent of the dairy cattle in the United States are affected with tuberculosis impresses me as a very conservative estimate. In New York State, about thirty-three per cent of all cattle tested were found to be tuberculous." Dr. Julius Rosenberg, of New York City, writes: "Cattle tuberculosis is rapidly increasing. There is scarcely a dairy herd without a number of infected animals. It is an ever growing menace. The health department of Boston estimates the percentage of tuberculous animals producing the city's milk supply to be from twenty to twenty-five per cent. Conservative estimate places the number of cows dying yearly from tuberculosis at one million, were they permitted to die a natural death; but they are killed before drawing the last gasp, and served as prime beef." In one year in the United States, the entire carcasses of thirty-five thousand one hundred three cattle were condemned because of generalized tuberculosis. In the same year, a portion of the carcass of ninety-nine thousand seven hundred thirty-nine more were rejected because of local tuberculosis.

Professor Ravenal, of the University of Wisconsin, says that of the thirty-five million hogs killed for food annually in the United States, seven million are found to be infected with tuberculosis. Some one has said that meat would sell for a dollar a pound if all the diseased meat were eliminated.

Ulcer of the stomach is one of our most common diseases. Leading surgeons have shown that it is ten times as frequent as was formerly supposed. It is clearly of dietetic origin, and is usually associated with too high consumption of protein, and especially of meat. Starches, sugars, and fats are not digested in the stomach, and require no acid. Proteins, on the other hand, are digested within the stomach, and require for their digestion a high percentage of hydrochloric acid. The excessive production of acid within the stomach, stimulated by too much protein, is probably the chief cause of the formation of ulcers. In 1908, Dr. Fenton B. Turck, of Chicago, said before the American Medical Association: "Ulcer of the stomach is not found in those countries where the inhabitants eat rice. It is evidently a meat eater's disease. The zone of ulcer is in the meat eater's zone."

Cancer is a disease of modern civilization. It is the one major unsolved problem in the field of medical science to-day. From the *Journal of the American Medical Association* of June 14, 1913, we quote: "That cancer has increased in recent years is perhaps a commonplace, but the extent of the increase is not generally realized. Under existing conditions, one in seven women and one in eleven men die of cancer." In the *Medical Record*, issue of May 15, 1915, Dr. W. G. Mayo is quoted as saying: "Cancer of the stomach forms nearly one third of all cancers of the human body.... Is it not possible that there is something in the habits of civilized man, in the cooking or other preparation of his food, which acts to produce the precancerous condition?... Within the last one hundred years, four times as much meat is taken as before that time. If flesh foods are not fully broken up, decomposition results, and active poisons are thrown into an organ not intended for their reception, and which has not had time to adapt itself to the new function."

Dr. L. Duncan Bulkley, senior physician to the New York Skin and Cancer Hospital, says on this point, "Analyzing the various data obtained, we find that cancer has increased in proportion to the consumption of four articles, meat, coffee, tea, and alcohol."

One is hardly up to date who does not present an abdominal scar caused by an offending appendix. At the fifteenth International Congress of Hygiene and Demography held in Washington, D. C., Dr. Henning contributed a paper dealing with "statistics upon the increase of appendicitis and its causes." He said: "A meat diet is of great influence in the development of appendicitis. This diet leads to constipation. In most instances, too long retention of intestinal contents in the cæcum causes slight inflammation in that region, the results of which are to weaken the appendix, and to render it nonresistant against later infection." When Dr. Lorenz, the celebrated Vienna surgeon, was in the United States, he called attention to the relatively greater prevalence of appendicitis in this country as compared with

Europe, and attributed it to the greater consumption of cold storage meats here, which he said rendered Americans unduly septic, and especially prone to infection of the appendix. Nicholas Senn was told by the hospital surgeons in Africa that they had never seen a case of appendicitis in a vegetable-eating African.

7. Trichinæ and Tapeworms

"A story is told of two of the most noted of Germans,—Bismarck, the statesman, and Virchow, the scientist. The latter had severely criticized the former in his capacity as chancellor, and was challenged to fight a duel. The man of science was found by Bismarck's seconds in his laboratory, hard at work at experiments which had for their object the discovery of a means of destroying trichinæ, then making ravages among animals in Germany. 'Ah,' said the doctor, 'a challenge from Prince Bismarck, eh? Well, well, as I am the challenged party, I suppose I have the choice of weapons. Here they are.' He held up two large sausages, which appeared to be exactly alike. 'One of these sausages,' he said, 'is filled with trichinæ. It is deadly. The other is perfectly wholesome. Externally, they can't be told apart. Let his excellency do me the honor to choose whichever of these he wishes and eat it, and I will eat the other.' No duel was fought, and no one accused Virchow of cowardice."

The trichina is a small, wormlike parasite found in the flesh of "measly pork," which, when eaten, burrows in the muscles of the human, producing an extremely painful and often fatal affection. About two per cent of hogs, it is estimated, harbor this parasite.

Practically speaking, the human being becomes the host of a tapeworm only by eating underdone flesh containing the larvæ of the parasite. (Thoroughly boiled or fried tapeworm is a harmless diet.) The ox, the hog, and the fish frequently harbor the larvæ of tapeworms.

8. Poor Economy

In these days of increased destruction and decreased production of human foods, it is of great importance to know how to secure a maximum amount of nutrition from a minimum expenditure of money. The world is facing a food shortage that in some places has assumed the proportion of the gaunt specter of famine. In view of this fact, it is well to remember that flesh is the most costly source of food. Sixty-two per cent of the best beefsteak is water. Flesh foods contain but twenty-five per cent nourishment, and seventy-five per cent waste matter. The grains contain seventy-five per cent nourishment, and but twenty-five per cent waste. Now it does not require a knowledge of higher mathematics to determine that since ten pounds of grain, when fed to an animal, make but one pound of flesh, the latter becomes a very costly source of our food supply.

9. The Testimony of Anatomy and Physiology

Even a kindergarten study of the structure of the human body reveals the fact that man was not intended to be a carnivorous, a herbivorous, or an omnivorous animal, but rather a frugivorous creature. He does not possess the rough, raspy tongue of the cat family, the long, pointed canine teeth of the lion, the sharp claws of the tiger, or the talons and hooked beak of the eagle. In the carnivora, the alimentary canal is very short, being only three times the length of the body. In herbivora, as the sheep, it is thirty times the length of the body. In frugivora, such as apes, monkeys, and man, it is twelve times the body length. Baron Cuvier, a famous anatomist, writes, "The natural food of man, judging from his structure, appears to consist principally of the fruits, roots, and other succulent parts of vegetables."

10. Flesh and Morals

The menu provided for man in the beginning did not include animal food. Not until one thousand six hundred fifty-six years of human history had passed was man permitted to eat flesh, and then only after every green thing had been destroyed by the Deluge. What we eat exercises a profound influence upon what we are, how we think, and how we feel. Let us divide the animal kingdom on the basis of diet and disposition. On the one hand, we have the lion, the tiger, the wolf, the bear, the leopard, the panther, etc.; all these are vicious, snarly, crabbed, ferocious beasts. What comprises their diet? We call them "beasts of prey." They feast upon the bloody, quivering flesh of their victims. On the other hand, we might mention the horse, the ox, the deer, the sheep, the elephant. Think of their dispositions, calm, quiet, pacific, easily domesticated. May it not be that their diet of cereals and herbs contributes to their peaceful temperament?

Dr. Curtis, the eminent physician to Mr. Garfield, said, "What parent is there who has not viewed with alarm how old Adam enters into the baby along with the first spoonful of chopped beef!" Gautier said, on this point: "The vegetarian régime, modified by the addition of milk, of fat of butter, of eggs, has great advantage. It adds to the alkalinity of the blood, accelerates oxidation, diminishes organic wastes and toxins. It exposes one much less likely than the ordinary régime to skin maladies, to arthritis, to congestions of internal organs. This régime tends to make us pacific beings, and not aggressive and violent."

To these we may add the testimony of Holy Writ, "Be not among winebibbers; among riotous eaters of flesh."

PHYSICAL BENEFITS OF JOY

he emotion of joy finds physiologic manifestations exactly opposite to those of sorrow and grief. There is increase of function in the muscles, and expansion of the blood vessels. As a result of increased muscular activity, the joyful person feels light and springy. Children, when joyful, dance and skip and clap their hands. The expansion of the blood vessels brings the "flush of joy." This increase in the circulation causes increased secretion of the digestive juices, with increased appetite, and increased power of digestion and absorption. This means increased nourishment. "Laugh and grow fat" has a physiologic basis. Fat people are not good-natured because they are fat, but they are fat because they are good-natured.

Laughter has a wonderfully beneficial influence on bodily functions—a fact recognized centuries ago when the wise man said, "A merry heart doeth good like a medicine." Laughter is a potent stimulant to all the helpful bodily functions. It hastens digestion, stimulates circulatory reaction, promotes tissue changes, enhances glandular activity, facilitates elimination, and altogether radiates a most beneficent influence throughout the body. Laugh, and the whole body laughs, and counts its work a pleasure.—*Dr. George A. Thomason.*

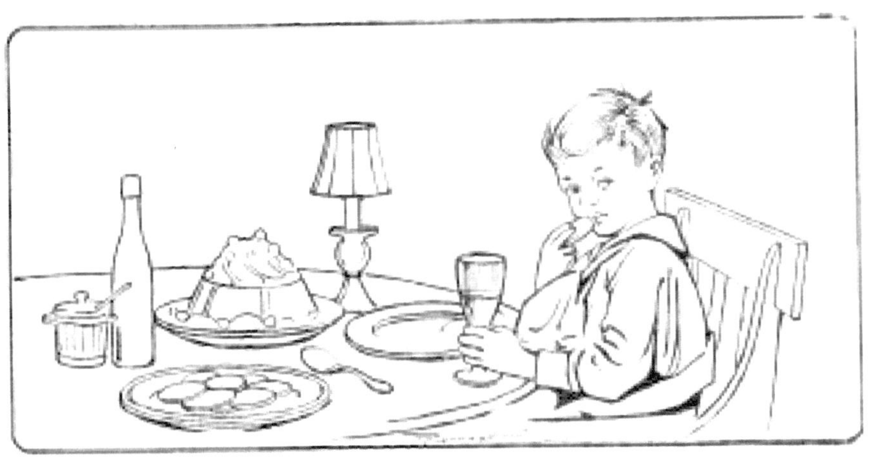

STIMULANTS AND CONDIMENTS

BY
ARTHUR N. DONALDSON, A.B., M.D.
*of the Faculty of the College of Medical
Evangelists, Loma Linda, California*

The Creator intended that the process of eating should be enjoyed. He has gathered the tasteless, insipid food elements together, and mixing in mineral and organic accessories, has produced for the tickling of our palates all the numberless flavors that the combined action of those highly specialized organs of taste and smell have enabled us to enjoy. The tasteless starch is bound up in the palatable potato; the insipid protein, in the pea, the lentil, and the bean; the rather nauseating fat, in the plump, appetizing olive. To the child not yet educated to the perverted demands of his father's palate, the thought, taste, and smell of these aromatic and savory substances produces a desire to eat. By the time he is twenty, he will not be satisfied with the natural flavor of his food. The cook must pepper or ginger it up, and he must further mustard or Worcestershire it to get it down. His soups are hot, and his salads are hotter. The palatable pleasure in a meal of his childhood is a lost asset. What has brought about this change in the appetite of man?

We all know, from experience, that we handle our food better if we relish it. This is due largely to the fact that the taste organs telegraph ahead to the stomach to prepare for work. The stomach responds by pouring out some digestive juices, and is consequently all ready to begin business the instant the tourist arrives. But when the food is bolted, there is a failure on the part of the taste nerves to telegraph ahead, unless they are stimulated more intensely by the addition of some readily diffusible sapid substance. Are we thus fooling nature?—We are not. Primarily, this unnatural stimulation leads to the most prevalent American dietetic sin; namely, overeating. We do not know when we have had enough. Dr. Wiggers, of Cornell University, has shown that overeating results in the surcharging of the blood stream with elements of digestion; and this, through the operation of physical laws, ultimately leads to arteriosclerosis and its chain of disasters. Secondly, with this unnatural stimulation of the taste nerves, the telegraphic messages to the stomach and the intestine are unreliable. Normally the tract is informed as to the nature of the food about to come, and is thus enabled to pour out a specific juice for a specific kind of food. Obviously this specificity which characterizes all normal processes is broken down, and the digestive function is placed under a handicap, when we cover up the natural taste with condiments.

The idea that condiments and stimulants act favorably in directly stimulating the production of gastric juice and in increasing gastric motor activity, and thus facilitating the digestive process, is a delusion. Professor Carlson, of Chicago University, has shown that these so-called stomachics and appetizers will have done their bit ere they enter the misunderstood stomach. And, our savory sauces and peppers being irritants in the mouth, they are no less irritants to the lining membrane of the stomach. They are always taboo in mild dyspeptic disorders, yet we think them just the appetizers for the run down nervous individual who never enjoys the pangs of hunger. Rather, he should be advised to oxygenate his impoverished blood by a brisk walk, to stir up his eliminative organs by vigorous exercise and the ingestion of water; for these bring no gastric catarrh, no sluggish liver.

It is recognized by every writer on dietetics, that condiments are irritating to the organs of elimination. The kidneys suffer, the ureters suffer, the bladder suffers, and the urethra suffers. We are very quick to stop the use of these substances when the kidneys give evidence of disease, and we will with alacrity drop the hot stuff from our dietary when the bladder and the urethra are inflamed. We do not like the smarting, burning pain produced by their presence. If they are detrimental during disease processes, they are just as detrimental in health. The long continued use of minute quantities of an irritant will incontrovertibly give ultimate evidence of its harmful nature, and we may expect such pathology as congestion of the liver, catarrh of the alimentary tract, hemorrhoids, nephritis, and general nutritive disturbances to be the possible heritage of our stimulating diet.

It is an interesting scientific fact that the highly soluble substances which are used as foods or food accessories are always irritating to the living membranes, particularly to the mucous membranes of the digestive organs with which they come in contact in the process of digestion, whether these membranes are healthy or diseased. Among such substances, we may mention sugar and salt.

Sugar and salt are excellent examples of the sapid, readily diffusible condiment so essential to our table, yet so invariably used to excess. We need about two teaspoonfuls of common salt a day—especially those who enjoy the vegetarian diet. Most vegetables are rich in potassium. This inorganic substance combines with sodium chloride, and is eliminated from the body. Consequently, the greater the amount of potassium in our food, the greater will be the loss of sodium chloride from the blood and the tissues, where it is an essential element, with the resultant need of an increased supply in our diet. Where there is an insufficient use of salt, there is a manifest disinclination to partake of the large variety of earth's products rich in potassium. But we are accustomed to the use of far more salt with our food than is necessary; and in excess, it is positively harmful, and the results of its use are serious.

Sugar is a pure carbohydrate; yet, by reason of its nature and use, it must be classed as a condiment. It, too, when used freely, brings on gastrointestinal catarrh through its direct irritant action, and affords unexcelled media for the growth of intestinal flora.

Stimulants

There are practically four strong stimulants to which civilized people are addicted; namely, alcohol, tobacco, tea, and coffee. Of the action of all, it may be said that the fatigue of nerve and brain is soothed by a spur. That is the work of a stimulant,—to goad the worn system to added effort, to produce an abnormal, false energy. Thus the individual is led on to a state of actual exhaustion without a warning note from his fatigued system. His energy is actually dissipated rather than increased. The results are shown in his heart, his nervous system, and his eliminative organs. Admiral Peary, speaking of the use of coffee in the rations of polar explorers, states that with the added effect of intense cold, it so stimulates the nerves as to cause the men to exhaust themselves, and soon wear out, by doing more than they can endure.

The actual extent of injury from the moderate use of tea and coffee has not been scientifically determined. The difficulty is, as Irving Fisher states it, "Sensitive people do not keep moderate." A little unnatural stimulation calls for a little more, and the tendency is to create a demand for something stronger. Fisher has truthfully declared that to abstain is much easier than to be moderate.

The claim that alcoholic beverages give added strength is a fallacy. The narcotic action of alcohol benumbs the sense of fatigue. From reliable clinical and laboratory findings, we are warranted in asserting with authority that alcohol lowers the power of all mental processes. The muscular efficiency is reduced. The ability of the body to protect itself against disease is undermined. The policemen of the body—the white corpuscles—are rendered more or less inactive—paralyzed; and the formation of other resistive elements of the blood is restricted. In other words, vital resistance is below par. Alcohol is furthermore a heart and circulatory depressant, and is no longer used by competent physicians as a circulatory stimulant. In short, it lowers mental and physical efficiency, and of course will naturally give its stamp to the unfortunate offspring.

Tobacco, too, blunts the edge of fatigue and worry. But its effect is transient, and the stimulation is followed by depression, which of course calls for more of the stimulant. Statistics tell us that where the weed is prohibited, efficiency is increased, and morale is improved.

Among the serious consequences of smoking, we find cancer of lip, tongue, and mouth, and serious cardiovascular changes. In a series of one hundred cases of cancer of the tongue and mouth, Dr. Abbe, of New York, found that ninety were inveterate users of tobacco; and he gives the stimulant the credit of being the ætiological factor in a high percentage of all malignant growths in this region. Tobacco not only directly affects the heart muscle, but its nicotine, through stimulation of the suprarenal gland, causes the production and throwing into the blood of an excessive amount of adrenalin, which brings about a tremendous rise in blood pressure, and of course an increase in the burden that the heart must carry. The ultimate result is arteriosclerosis, tobacco heart, nephritis, and very possibly a closing of the scene with a paralytic stroke.

Professor Fisher very aptly appeals against the introduction of more poisons into a system already burdened with poisons of its own elaboration.

We are not at liberty to ignore nature and her laws. Our bodies are not our own. When the Creator has opened to us of heaven's abundance for the sustenance of life, and has given us a dietary that answers every need of palate and body, we are palpably in error before our Maker when we question His wisdom, and take into our systems those substances which we know to be destructive to mind, soul, and body.

> OUR country, however, is blessed with an abundance of foodstuffs; and if our people will economize in their use of food, providently confining themselves to the quantities required for the maintenance of health and strength, if they will eliminate waste, and if they will make use of those commodities of which we have a surplus, and thus free for export a larger proportion of those required by the world now dependent on us, we shall not only be able to accomplish our obligations to them, but we shall obtain and establish reasonable prices at home. — *Woodrow Wilson.*

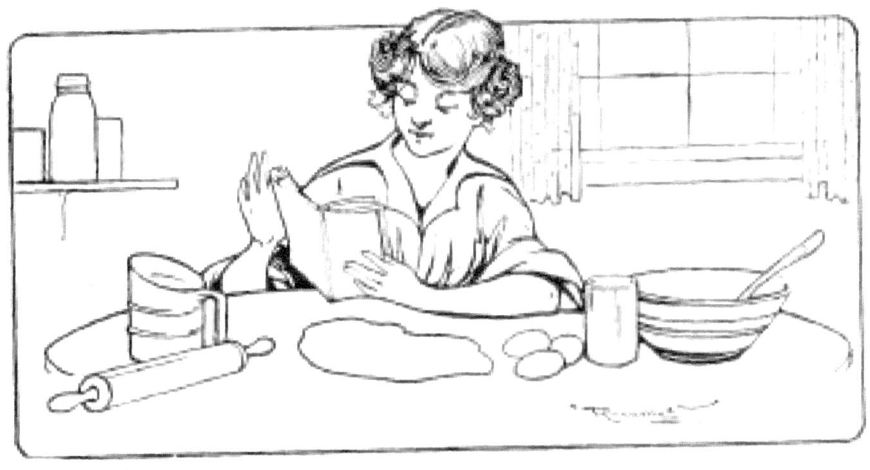

SIMPLE MENUS AND RECIPES
BY
MR. H. S. ANDERSON

Food Specialist, College of Medical Evangelists and
Loma Linda Sanitarium

The art of planning and combining the food for a meal is of no small importance to the housewife or the cook. The very best foods may be served in such combinations as to bring distress to the digestive organs, and produce weakness instead of strength.

Because human beings differ so much, and their needs are so varied, it is impossible to lay down any set of rules on diet alike for all. There are general principles, however, by which all may be guided, and which, if heeded, can accomplish more for the individual or the family, in maintaining health, than all doctors' prescriptions. This is made plain by the fact that it is better to know how to keep well than how to cure disease.

It is therefore of great importance for those who have the responsibility of planning for the table, to have a working knowledge of the principles which guide in making out a balanced menu.

In the planning of a meal, careful study should be given to the combination of foods. On the one hand, only such foods as digest well together should be used at one meal. On the other hand, foods should be chosen that will supply all the needed elements in about the right proportion.

Because of the woody substances found in vegetables, especially the coarse or fibrous vegetables, such as carrots, beets, turnips, cabbage, potatoes, and others, they digest slowly, and consequently remain a long time in the stomach before they are broken sufficiently for intestinal digestion. Fruits remain in the stomach a short time, and, owing to the large amount of saccharine matter they contain, are apt to ferment if retained too long.

Fruit and vegetables therefore should not be eaten at the same meal. This has special reference to the coarse and underground vegetables; while the finer or fruity vegetables, such as green peas, corn, squash, tomatoes, etc., and some others which also ripen in the sun, may be used with almost any food.

A safe rule in planning a meal, is to be sure that the *soup*, the *relishes* (greens, salads, etc.), and the *dessert*, if used, combine well together, as these are so generally used by nearly all classes of people when placed on the menu. Then if fruit is used, in salad, or as dessert, there should be on the menu at least one of the finer vegetables, such as tomatoes, corn, or the like, which can be eaten with the fruit; and if the meal is planned without fruit, any of the coarser vegetables may be used as desired.

A large variety should not be planned for any one meal. It is a great additional expense; and besides, when several articles are taken at one meal, fermentation is likely to occur and the system will not be so well nourished. Recent research work has shown that the digestive juices vary both in kind and in quantity with different kinds of food eaten. This may explain why many persons cannot digest complex mixtures and extensive variety, and is a mighty argument for simplicity at meal-time.

A select variety, of only a few kinds of food, at any one meal, with diversity in the meals from day to day, will prove advantageous to the individual and the family, both from the standpoint of economy, and from the health point of view.

An excess of milk and sugar taken together clogs the system, and should be avoided. Fats are more digestible cold than hot, because hot fat tends to coat and intimately penetrate the food with which it is cooked. This is especially true of fried foods, part of the food being surrounded with a layer of fat, keeping the digestive juices from acting on the other food elements. When subjected to a high temperature, fats decompose, and the resulting acids are very irritating to the mucous membranes of the stomach and the intestines.

The following combinations of food digest well together:

- Grains, fruits, and nuts
- Grains with milk
- Grains with eggs
- Grains, vegetables, and nuts

Foods that do not digest well together are:

- Milk and sugar taken together, in large quantities
- Fruit and vegetables
- Foods cooked in fats

A balanced dietary is one that supplies in about the right proportion all the kinds of food required to nourish the body. From the earliest impressions of childhood, many persons have received the idea that the most important article of diet is animal flesh. In most cases, this idea has been accepted without question or thought, and probably has never been challenged. A careful study of the subject, however, will show that with the use of meat, there is great danger of an excess of protein above the minimum requirements, there being thus placed upon the liver and the kidneys an amount of work which should not be imposed on these vitally important organs.

To combine foods in such a way as to supply all the needed elements, we should choose something from each of the different classes of food elements. There should also be among these such as supply sufficient cellulose and mineral. To illustrate this point, a few menus will be given that are extremely unbalanced, or one-sided, that we may understand more forcibly, by contrast, what a good meal is:

1. Soy bean soup Lentil patties Cottage cheese Custard pie Milk	Too much building food Too concentrated Too little bulk
2. White rice Mashed potato Spaghetti White crackers Butter Cake	Too much fuel food Too little bulk and mineral Lacks building food (protein)
3. Vegetable soup Wax beans Lettuce Stewed beets Bran biscuit Strawberries	Too little building food Too little fuel food Too bulky Lacking in nourishment Bad combination

In order to make a balanced meal out of the above foods, it would be necessary to choose something from each of these unbalanced meals, and it would not be necessary to choose a large variety in order to supply the needs of the body. Upon examination, we find that bread (entire wheat) possesses properties which so nearly represent the constituent parts of the body as to make such bread ideal for the building up and keeping in repair of the human body. In the matter of building food (protein), bread contains about ten per cent, or about the recognized dietary requirement.

Bread is an exceedingly digestible food; and experiments taken as a whole show nearly ninety-eight per cent of the starch, or carbohydrate nutrients, and about eighty-eight per cent of the gluten, or protein constituents, assimilated by the body. See Snyder's "Human Foods," page 179; also table, page 23.

Many other grains, such as corn, oats, rye, barley, and rice, all contain heat-

and energy-producing substances and tissue-forming elements in about the right proportion to meet the needs of the body. Exception is made of rice, which is slightly deficient in protein.

Bread of some kind, therefore, is the "backbone" of the meal. Around it are grouped the various fruits and vegetables for change and variety, alternating with one of the more solid foods, rich in protein, such as cottage cheese, eggs, nuts, or any of the various legumes, as peas, beans, lentils, etc. Of all the legumes, the soy bean takes the lead for building food, containing nearly twice the per cent of protein found in round steak. These more hearty foods should be used with discretion, especially during the summer months, when well baked breads, fruits, and green garden products constitute the ideal diet.

Potatoes, which are mostly starch, and eggs, which are largely albumen and fat, may be combined in such a way as to furnish all the needed elements in the right proportion. As rice is nearly all starch, and beans are rich in protein, these make an excellent combination. Nuts, rich in proteins and fats, and fruits, containing sugars and acids, also make an ideal combination. To a meal composed largely of rice and potatoes, which are deficient in fats, there may be added a little cream, a few ripe olives, a few nuts, or an egg, to give a well balanced ration.

The custom of eating a light lunch at noon, and reserving the heaviest meal for the close of the day, while actuated to a great extent by seeming necessities, or convenience, is not, as a rule, found a benefit to health. As a result of a hearty meal at night, the digestive process is continued through the sleeping hours; and though the stomach works constantly, its work is not properly accomplished. The sleep is often disturbed by unpleasant dreams; and in the morning, the person awakes unrefreshed, and with little relish for breakfast.

The practice of eating but two meals a day is generally found a benefit to health; yet under some circumstances, persons may require a third meal. This should, however, if taken at all, be very light, and of foods very easily digested, so that when we lie down to rest, the stomach may have its work all done, and it, as well as the other organs of the body, may enjoy rest.

In the following menus, some allowance is made for variety. Some persons will not require everything named on the menu; and each person will choose such things, and in such amounts, as experience and sound judgment prove to be best suited to his own necessities.

MENUS FOR ONE WEEK

SUNDAY

Breakfast

STEAMED NATURAL RICE		CREAM PEAS ON TOAST	
STRAWBERRIES	CORN BREAD	MILK	VEGETABLE BUTTER

Dinner

ENTIRE WHEAT BREAD	BEANS WITH NOODLES

LETTUCE   CORN ON COB   CLUSTER   BUTTER
                                  RAISINS

Luncheon

CREAMED RICE   CORN MEAL CRISPS   ZWIEBACK

PEACH SAUCE   CEREAL COFFEE

Steamed Rice.—Wash one cup of natural brown rice, and put to cook in three cups of boiling water. Let boil gently until the water is absorbed and the rice looks dry; then set on the edge of the stove, well covered, to steam for fifteen minutes.

Cream Peas on Toast.—One cup drained green peas, one third cup water, three tablespoonfuls rich cream, salt. Bring the water and the peas to a boil, mash through a colander to remove the hulls, and season with cream and salt. Dip a slice of zwieback into hot milk to soften, lay on a platter, cover with a spoonful of the cream of peas, and serve.

Corn Bread.—One and one third cups corn meal, two tablespoonfuls whole wheat flour, two and one half tablespoonfuls vegetable butter, two tablespoonfuls brown sugar, one and one fourth teaspoonfuls salt, one and one third cups boiling water, two eggs. Mix all the dry ingredients in a bowl. Add the butter, and pour on the boiling water in a *slow* stream, stirring while it is being poured in. Add two or three tablespoonfuls of cold water if needed to make a medium batter. Separate the eggs, and beat the whites stiff. Beat the yolks, and fold them into the whites. Add the corn mixture, and mix, using the folding motion. Pour into an oiled shallow baking pan, and bake in a quick oven.

Butter Substitutes

Owing to the great increase in disease among animals, and along with this, the advance in prices of nearly all foodstuffs, a desire has been created for some substitute for dairy butter, which would prove both wholesome and appetizing. The following butter substitutes are now used to some extent both for cooking and for table use, and are easily prepared:

Emulsified Vegetable Oil.—Secure a high grade cottonseed, corn, or peanut oil. Beat one egg slightly, then add the oil in a very slow stream at first, beating continuously, and increase as the egg takes up the oil. Add two teaspoonfuls lemon juice, then more oil, until three cupfuls have been used, and the mixture is smooth and thick. Salt to taste, put into a well covered jar, and use the same as butter.

Vegetable Butter.—Take three cupfuls of any good coconut product on the market, such as kokofat or kaola, or a good brand of hydrogenated vegetable fat, as crisco.[1] Add the juice of half a lemon, salt to taste, and a few drops of vegetable butter color. Mix with a spoon until the color of dairy butter. The juice from carrots, grated and pressed, may be used instead of the lemon juice and the butter

---

[1] Note.—The presence of a proprietary substance in a recipe must not be understood as guarantee by the authors. We know very little regarding the manufacture of the above named products; but we have reason to believe they are wholesome, and contain no animal products.

color if desired.

In harmony with the recent food pledge, saying, "Use no butter in cooking," all the recipes in these menus are prepared without the use of dairy butter. However, the same recipes may be prepared with dairy butter instead of the vegetable fats if so desired.

Beans with Noodles. —Wash one cup navy or Lima beans, add three cups water and a little salt, and let boil gently until tender. Beat one egg slightly, with two teaspoonfuls of water or milk and a pinch of salt. Add one cup of pastry flour, or enough to make a stiff dough. Knead well, and divide into two pieces. Roll out into thin sheets about the thickness of paper, having the dough well floured. Let dry a few minutes, then cut into strips about two inches wide. Lay in tiers, and shred very fine with a sharp knife. Drain the liquid from the beans, add to it enough water to make three cups of liquid, and add salt to taste. Add two teaspoonfuls of vegetable butter, and bring to a boil. Sprinkle the noodles into the boiling broth, and let cook gently for fifteen minutes. Add the cooked beans, and shake together, reheat, and serve. New peas may be substituted for beans when in season.

Corn on Cob. —Husk full ears of corn, and brush off the silks with a stiff brush. Wash, and drop into boiling water to which has been added a little milk or lemon juice. Bring to a good boil; then draw the saucepan to one side of the stove, and let simmer for twenty minutes.

Entire Wheat Bread. —Three cups warm water, one half cake compressed yeast, three tablespoonfuls brown sugar, two tablespoonfuls vegetable fat, one tablespoonful salt, seven cups entire wheat flour. Dissolve the yeast in two teaspoonfuls of water, add the liquid, and mix all the ingredients to a medium *soft* dough. Turn out on a slightly floured board, and knead until elastic to the touch; then return to an oiled bowl, cover, and let stand in a warm room to rise until, when tapped sharply, it *begins* to sink (about two hours). Work down well, turn over in the bowl, and let rest until it begins to rise again (about fifteen minutes); then mold into loaves, and put into pans for baking. Brush over the top of each loaf with an oiled brush, and let rise until half again its original bulk; then bake in a good oven. These coarse breads must be watched closer during the rising than those made from white flour, as they get light in much less time.

Creamed Rice. —Heat some milk in a double boiler, and when it is hot, add enough cooked rice to have it creamy, but not too soft. Add a pinch of salt, and a little rich cream, if you have it at hand, and serve.

Corn Meal Crisps. —One cup white corn meal, one cup pastry flour, one half teaspoonful salt, one tablespoonful brown sugar, two tablespoonfuls vegetable fat, scant one half cup water. Mix all the dry ingredients, add the oil, and rub between the hands to distribute the fat through the grain. Add the water, and mix to a dough. Roll out to a thickness of one fourth of an inch, cut with a biscuit cutter, prick with a fork, and bake in a hot oven, to a light brown.

Zwieback. —Cut stale bread into slices about one half inch thick. Lay these in a baking pan, and put them into the warming oven until the moisture is evaporated; then put them into a hot oven until they are a light brown all the way through.

MONDAY

Breakfast

CREAM	SCRAMBLED EGG WITH NEW TOMATO	BUTTER
WHEAT PUFFS	STEAMED PEARL BARLEY	STEWED PRUNES

Dinner

SLICED TOMATO	FARMER'S FAVORITE SOUP	SPINACH
ROASTED POTATO WITH DRESSING	EGG GRAVY BUTTER	RYE BREAD

Luncheon

BAKED BANANA	TOMATO SANDWICHES	BLACKBERRIES
RYE BISCUIT	MILK	CRACKERS

Steamed Pearl Barley.—Wash one cup pearl barley, and put to cook in four cups boiling water. Add one fourth teaspoonful salt, and let boil gently until the water is absorbed and the grain looks dry; then cover, and set on the edge of the stove to steam for forty minutes. This grain is preferably cooked on a hot stone in the fireless.

Scrambled Egg with New Tomato.—Rub a large ripe tomato with the back of a knife; then remove the skin, and cut the tomato into pieces. Put it into a small pan, with one teaspoonful vegetable butter and a pinch of salt, and bring to a boil. Break two eggs slightly with a fork, put them into a hot oiled frying pan, and stir until they are soft scrambled. Have the tomato drained, add the pulp to the scrambled eggs, and mix, being careful not to cook the egg too much. Serve on toast.

Wheat Puffs.—One and one fourth cups sifted pastry flour, one fourth cup whole wheat flour, two teaspoonfuls melted vegetable butter, one fourth teaspoon salt, one cup milk, one egg. Make a batter of the flour, the salt, the milk, the egg yolk, and the butter, and stir smooth. Beat the white stiff, and pour the batter into the beaten white, mixing as it is being poured in, and using the folding motion, so as not to break down the lightness of the egg. Pour into hot oiled iron gem pans, and bake in a quick oven.

Stewed Prunes.—Wash dried prunes thoroughly, and let them soak overnight. Then bring them to a boil, and let simmer for two hours or more, and they will need no sweetening.

Farmer's Favorite Soup.—One half cup rich sour cream, one third cup macaroni, one small onion, one stalk celery, one small carrot, one medium sized potato, chopped parsley, salt. Drop the macaroni into three cupfuls boiling salted water, and cook until thoroughly done. Have the vegetables cut into small dice. Put the cream into a small pan, and stir over the fire until the oil separates, and the albumen turns a light brown color. The degree of browning determines the flavor of the soup. Add the diced onion, carrot, and celery, and stir for a few moments. Add three cupfuls water, the diced potato, and a little salt, and cook until the vegetables are thoroughly done. Add the macaroni water to the vegetable soup; then lay the macaroni on a board, cut into small rings, and drop into the soup. Boil up well, add chopped parsley, and serve.

Roasted Potato.—Peel eight medium sized potatoes, and boil until they are about half done; then drain them, and save the water. Lay the potatoes in an oiled baking pan, brush with oil, sprinkle with salt and flour, and put into a hot oven to brown.

Baked Dressing.—Two cups soaked stale bread, one half cup milk, three table-spoonfuls chopped onion, one and one half tablespoonfuls vegetable butter, three tablespoonfuls browned flour, a pinch of sage and marjoram, and salt to taste. Soak the bread in cold water until it is soft all the way through, then press it out. Put the butter, the onion, and the savory into a small pan, and let them simmer for a few moments, to soften the onion, but do not brown. Add the brown flour, then the milk, and stir smooth. Add the bread, salt to taste, and mix. Bake in an oiled brick tin, or spread among the roasted potatoes when they are partly browned, and finish baking them together.

Egg Gravy.—Two tablespoonfuls vegetable fat, one teaspoonful chopped onion, three tablespoonfuls flour, one egg, one and one half cups potato water or almost any vegetable broth. Put the oil into a frying pan, and when it is quite hot, add the whole egg. Break the yolk with a fork, turn it over, and stir until brown over the entire surface. Remove the brown egg from the oil, and chop with a knife. Add the flour to the oil, and stir until a light brown. Add the onion, and stir; then the chopped egg and one third of the water, and stir smooth. Add the balance of the water, and boil up. Let simmer for ten minutes, and serve. The egg may be omitted, if desired; but without it, the gravy will have less flavor.

Spinach.—Wash the greens in several waters. If the spinach is young and tender, it can be cooked with no additional water beyond that remaining on the leaves after washing. As the spinach ages, it absorbs bitter flavor, and should then be cooked in boiling water, with the *cover off*. When done, drain, cut with a knife, season with salt and a little vegetable butter, reheat, and serve.

Rye Bread.—Two cups warm water, one half cake compressed yeast, one and one half tablespoonfuls vegetable fat, two tablespoonfuls brown sugar, two teaspoonfuls salt, four cups white bread flour, three cups rye flour. Dissolve the yeast in two teaspoonfuls water, add the liquid, and beat in three cups best bread flour to a smooth batter. Cover, and let stand in a warm room to rise for one and one half hours. Add the salt, the sugar, and the oil, and beat into the sponge. Mix in the rye flour and the remaining cup of white flour, to a medium dough. Knead on a board until elastic to the touch, then return to an oiled bowl, cover, and let rise the same as for entire wheat bread, in Sunday's lesson. When ready to mold into loaves, roll out six buns, and lay on an oiled pie tin, and let rise for *rye biscuit*. Divide the remaining dough into two parts, and roll out into the shape of ordinary rye bread loaves. Lay in an oiled baking pan, leaving space between. Brush with an oiled brush, and cut three gashes across each loaf with a sharp knife, and let rise until light, then bake in a quick oven.

Baked Banana.—Select firm, rather ripe bananas, put them into the oven without removing the skins, and bake until the skins burst. Then remove from the oven, and serve in a folded napkin.

Tomato Sandwiches.—Peel ripe tomatoes without scalding, by first scraping them with the back of a knife; then cut into thin slices. Cut bread into very thin slices, and spread one slice with butter, and the opposite slice with mayonnaise or boiled dressing. Lay tomatoes between the slices, cut in triangles, and serve.

TUESDAY

Breakfast

CANTALOUPE	SAVORY HASH	JELLIED EGG
MILK	CORN DODGERS	HONEY

Dinner

SLICED TOMATO	NEW ENGLAND DINNER	ENGLISH WAL-NUTS
ENTIRE WHEAT BREAD	BUTTER	CREAM RICE PUDDING

Luncheon

MILK TOAST	RAISIN SANDWICH	PEACH SAUCE
UNLEAVENED RYE WAFERS		WATERMELON

Savory Hash.—Two cups cold boiled potatoes cut in dice, three fourths cup of the baked dressing as given in Monday's lesson, cold, and cut into small dice, one and one half tablespoonfuls diced onion, one and one half tablespoonfuls vegetable butter, one tablespoonful brown flour, a pinch of sage or marjoram, one half cup milk, and salt to taste. Put the butter, the onion, and the savory into a small pan, and simmer for a few moments; then add the brown flour and a little of the milk, and stir smooth. Add the balance of the milk, and boil up. Salt to taste, and add the diced food. Sprinkle the diced potato with a little salt, add the gravy mixture, and mix with a fork. Put into an oiled baking pan, brush over the top with a little cream, and bake in a hot oven to a nice brown.

Jellied Egg.—Put one pint of water into a small, narrow saucepan, and bring to a boil. Drop in one egg with a spoon, and set the saucepan immediately on the table for from seven to eight minutes; then serve. If more eggs are added, the amount of water must be increased proportionately.

Corn Dodgers.—One cup corn meal (preferably toasted lightly in the oven), one and one half tablespoonfuls vegetable fat, one half teaspoonful salt, one tablespoonful brown sugar, one and one half cups boiling water. Mix all the dry ingredients, add the fat and pour on the boiling water and stir smooth. A few more tablespoonfuls water may be added if needed to make a batter of such a consistency as to drop from a spoon, but not run. Drop from the side of a spoon, onto an oiled baking pan, and bake in a quick oven.

Corn Cake.—Use the above recipe, and spread in an oiled baking pan one fourth inch deep, and bake in a hot oven.

New England Dinner.—Six medium small potatoes, four small carrots, four small turnips, six small onions, one half small cabbage, one and one half tablespoonfuls vegetable butter, and salt to taste. Quarter the peeled turnips and carrots. Add the onions whole, and put into a saucepan with water enough to cover the vegetables, and salt, and bring to a boil. Separate the cabbage leaves, and drop them into another vessel of boiling water, to blanch them for five minutes; then drain, and add to the boiling vegetables. Add the potatoes, and let boil gently until nearly done; then add the vegetable butter, and let simmer until thoroughly done.

Cream Rice Pudding.—One half cup uncooked white rice, five cupfuls milk, scant one third cup sugar, vanilla flavor. Wash the rice thoroughly, add the milk, and cook in a double boiler for three fourths of an hour. Add the sugar and the vanilla flavor, and pour into an oiled baking pan and bake in a moderate oven. As soon as the first crust forms, stir it down, at the same time stirring the rice. Then allow the last crust to form and brown, and remove from the oven.

Milk Toast.—Put a piece of zwieback into a bowl, pour scalding hot milk over it, and serve.

Raisin Sandwich.—Chop one half cup seeded raisins fine, and add one fourth cup ground walnuts. Add one and one half tablespoonfuls mayonnaise dressing and one teaspoonful lemon juice, and mix well. Spread between slices of thinly buttered bread, cut in triangles, and serve.

Rye Wafers.—One cup rye flour, one cup pastry flour, two and one half tablespoonfuls vegetable fat, two tablespoonfuls brown sugar, one half teaspoonful salt, one half cup water, or barely enough to mix to a stiff dough. Mix all the dry ingredients, add the oil, and rub the flour between the hands to distribute the oil evenly. Add the water very slowly, stirring meantime to avoid getting any part of the flour wet and sticky. Work on the board until mixed, then roll out to one fourth inch thickness, cut with a biscuit cutter, prick with a fork, and bake in a hot oven to a light brown.

Rye Sticks.—Take the above dough, roll out one half inch thick, cut into long strips about one third inch wide, then crosswise into three-inch lengths. Lay in a baking pan, leaving a little space between, and bake to a light brown color.

WEDNESDAY

Breakfast

STEWED CHERRIES	STEAMED WHEAT	PLAIN OMELET
CREAM	CORN MEAL PUFFS	BUTTER

Dinner

VEGETABLE JULIENNE SOUP	STRING BEANS	MACARONI	FAMILY STYLE

BUTTER RAISED CORN BREAD WATERMELON

Luncheon

WHEAT GRUEL STEWED PRUNES RYE STICKS

ZWIEBACK GRAPES MILK

Steamed Wheat.—Pick over one cup of wheat, and wash in several waters. Let soak overnight; then drain, add four cups boiling water, and let boil slowly until the water is evaporated and the wheat looks dry. Cover, and let stand on the edge of the stove to steam for forty minutes. This grain is best cooked on a hot stone in fireless overnight.

Plain Omelet.—One egg, one tablespoonful milk, a pinch of salt. Beat the yolk until thick, add the milk, and mix well. Add a pinch of salt to the white, and beat stiff. Fold the yolk into the white, and pour the mixture into a hot oiled fry pan, and set into the oven until just barely *set*. While still in the pan, turn one half of the omelet over the other half, by slipping a knife under one side and turning it over on the other section. Invert on a hot platter, and serve.

Corn Meal Puffs.—One cup pastry flour, one third cup corn meal, one half teaspoonful salt, two teaspoonfuls vegetable butter, one scant cup milk, one egg separated. Make a batter of the milk, the flour, the corn meal, the salt, the melted fat, and the egg yolk, and stir smooth. Beat the white stiff, and fold the batter into it. Pour into hot oiled iron gem pans, and bake in a quick oven.

Vegetable Julienne Soup.—One medium small potato, one small carrot, one small turnip, one stalk celery, one half cup cauliflowerlets or string beans, peas, or any fresh green vegetable, one small tomato, one teaspoonful vegetable butter, two cups cold water, two cups vegetable broth, salt to taste. Cut all the coarse vegetables into very thin shreds, and put into a small pan with the vegetable butter and one fourth cup water, and let simmer until the moisture is absorbed; then add the rest of the water, and boil up. Add the cut potato and tomato and the vegetable broth. Salt to taste, and let cook until the vegetables are thoroughly done. Add a sprinkle of chopped parsley, and serve.

Macaroni Family Style.—One cup macaroni raw, one cup tomato pulp, one tablespoonful vegetable butter, one tablespoonful chopped onion, a sprinkle of sage or thyme, one egg, and salt to taste. Break the macaroni into inch lengths, drop into salted boiling water, and let cook until thoroughly done; then drain in a colander. Put the butter, the onion, and the savory into a small pan, and simmer for a few moments, but do not brown. Add the tomato, bring to a boil, and salt to taste. Pour the hot sauce into the egg, stirring as it is being poured in. Add the cooked macaroni, pour all into an oiled baking pan, and bake to a light brown.

String Beans.—Select young and tender beans, string them, and break them into short lengths. Wash, and lift them out of the water; put into a saucepan with enough boiling water to cover the beans. Add salt, and let cook gently, having the cover drawn to one side of the saucepan. When done, add a little vegetable butter and serve. When the beans are aged, they should be lifted out of the water and put into a covered vessel containing a little hot vegetable oil, and stirred over the fire for ten minutes before the water is added to them; and when cooked, they will be very tender.

Raised Corn Bread. — In order to incorporate in corn bread enough moisture so that it will not dry out after baking, a certain proportion of the liquid used may be poured over the meal boiling hot; thus the needed moisture is absorbed before making into bread, as follows:

Three cups water, one half cake compressed yeast, four cups best bread flour, two cups corn meal, one tablespoon salt, three tablespoons sugar, two tablespoons vegetable fat. Sift the flour into a large bowl, and leave space at one side of the flour for the sponge. Dissolve the yeast in two teaspoons water, add one cup warm water, and pour on one side of the flour. Stir enough flour into this liquid to make a thin, smooth batter. Cover, and set in a warm room until light (about one and one half hours). Put the corn meal into a small bowl, and pour on gradually, in a slow stream, two cups boiling water, stirring as it is poured in, and let stand one half hour.

When the sponge is sufficiently light, add the salt, the sugar, and the vegetable fat, and mix well. Add the scalded and warm corn meal, and mix all into a soft dough. Turn out on a floured board, and knead until elastic to the touch. Then return to an oiled bowl, cover, let rise, and finish the same as for entire wheat bread.

Wheat Gruel. — Take the steamed wheat left over from breakfast, add water to cover, and let cook gently until well done. Mash through a strainer, season with salt and a little cream or canned milk, and serve.

Rye Sticks. — The recipe for rye sticks is given following the recipe for rye wafers in Tuesday's lesson.

THURSDAY

Breakfast

BUTTER	BAKED GARBANZOS WITH APPLE SAUCE	CREAM
GRANO CEREAL WITH DATES	ENTIRE WHEAT BREAD	

Dinner

SLICED TOMATO	NAVY BEAN SOUP ARMY STYLE	STEWED CARROTS
NOODLES AU GRATIN	RYE BREAD BUTTER	STEAMED RAISINS

Luncheon

NUT AND JELLY SANDWICHES

BANANA RICE	BUCKWHEAT STICKS	RHUBARB SAUCE

Grano Cereal. — Two cups pastry flour, one third cup rolled oats, one fourth cup corn meal, one fourth teaspoonful salt, large one half cup water. Mix all the dry ingredients, and add the water slowly, stirring constantly to a very stiff dough. Knead a few moments, then roll out one fourth inch thick. Cut into strips about three inches wide, prick with a fork, lay in a baking pan, and bake in a medium oven until a very light brown and fairly crisp. When cool, grind through a food chopper, using a coarse knife. Serve with milk or cream.

Grano with Dates.—Two cups water, one cup grano cereal, one half cup washed and pitted dates, a pinch of salt. Bring the water to a boil, and sprinkle in the grano. Stir until thick, then add the dates, and serve with cream.

Baked Garbanzos (chick peas).—Wash one cup garbanzos, and soak overnight. Drain, add two cups boiling water, and let boil gently until thoroughly done, or cook in fireless overnight. Return to the fire, add salt to taste, and let cook gently until the liquid is reduced; then put into the oven in a covered dish, and bake until they begin to brown slightly on the bottom.

Navy Bean Soup Army Style.—One cup navy beans, seven cups water, two thirds cup diced carrot, one third cup diced onion, one tablespoonful vegetable butter, salt to taste. Wash the beans, and cook very slowly until tender, adding the salt when they are about half done. Put the butter, the diced carrot, and the onion into a small pan with three tablespoonfuls water, and stir over the fire until the water is absorbed; then add to the bean soup, and let boil gently for thirty minutes or more. Add a sprinkle of chopped parsley, and serve.

Stewed Carrots.—Two cups sliced young carrots, one and one half cups hot water, two teaspoonfuls vegetable butter, one teaspoon flour, salt. Wash and scrape young carrots, and slice quite thin. Add the hot water, and salt to taste, and let cook gently until the liquid is reduced to one half cup. Rub the flour and the butter smooth in a small pan. Add one third of the liquid, and stir smooth. Add the balance of the liquid, and boil up. Add the carrots, reheat, and serve. A little rich cream or canned milk may be added if desired.

Noodles au Gratin.—Roll out and cut noodles the same as given in recipe for Sunday dinner. Sprinkle into boiling salted water, and cook the same as macaroni, or about fifteen minutes. Drain well, saving the liquid for gravies or sauces. Make a cream sauce by rubbing together in a saucepan two tablespoonfuls vegetable butter and two tablespoonfuls flour; then add one third cup hot milk, and stir smooth. Add two thirds cup more milk, boil up, and salt to taste. Add enough of the cream sauce to the noodles to flavor them and not have them too soft. Pour into an oiled baking pan, and grate fresh bread crumbs over the top, pressing them down with a spoon to moisten them. Sprinkle with cream or bits of butter, and bake to a nice brown.

Steamed Raisins.—Dip cluster raisins into water, drain, and lay between two pie tins; put into the oven until hot through; then serve.

Banana Rice.—Take the recipe for creamed rice as given in the lesson for Sunday evening luncheon. Slice one large banana, sprinkle with a little sugar, mix lightly into the hot creamed rice, and serve.

Nut and Jelly Sandwiches.—Add finely chopped or ground walnuts to jelly in the proportion to spread nicely on bread. Cut bread into very thin slices. Spread one slice with butter, and the opposite slice with the nut mixture. Fold together, cut in triangles, and serve.

Buckwheat Sticks.—One cup pastry flour, one cup buckwheat flour, one half teaspoonful salt, two and one half tablespoonfuls vegetable fat, two tablespoonfuls brown sugar, scant one half cup water, or barely enough to mix the flour to a stiff dough. Mix all the dry ingredients, add the fat, and rub between hands to distribute the oil evenly. Add the water very slowly, stirring meantime; and as soon as the flour can be worked together by sufficient moisture, lay on the board, and work for a few moments; then roll out to one third inch thickness. Cut into strips one third inch in width, then crosswise into sticks three inches long. Lay in a baking pan, leaving a little space between, and bake to a very light brown.

Buckwheat Wafers.—Take the above dough, roll out one fourth inch thick, cut with a biscuit cutter, prick with a fork, and bake the same as sticks.

FRIDAY

Breakfast

POACHED EGG	CORN MEAL WITH RAISINS	CANTALOUPE
CREAM	BAKED POTATO RYE BREAD	BUTTER

Dinner

CUCUMBERS	CREAM OF TOMATO SOUP	STEWED CORN
VEGETABLE LOAF	COUNTRY GRAVY BUTTER	ENTIRE WHEAT BREAD

Luncheon

FRUIT SOUP	CORN FLAKES CREAM	BUCKWHEAT WAFERS
WATERMELON	APPLES	ZWIEBACK

Corn Meal with Raisins.—Wash one half cup raisins, and put them between two pie tins in the oven until hot through. Put one cup corn meal into a baking pan, and toast lightly in the oven; then sprinkle it gradually into three and one half cupfuls of boiling water, with one fourth teaspoonful salt, and let cook gently for ten minutes. Add the raisins, let cook for twenty minutes more, and serve.

Poached Egg.—Bring water to a boil in a saucepan, break the egg into a separate dish, and drop carefully into the boiling water. Set immediately to one side of the stove until the egg is firm enough to remove, and the white will be tender and jellylike.

Cream of Tomato Soup.—Two cupfuls strained tomato, one cupful water, two teaspoonfuls vegetable butter, one tablespoonful light brown flour, one cupful canned milk or rich cream, salt to taste. Bring the water, the tomato, and the butter to a boil. Thicken with the flour made smooth with a little cold water. Salt to taste, add canned milk (unheated), strain, and serve. If cream is used, omit the butter.

Vegetable Loaf.—One and one half cups soaked stale bread, three fourths cup cooked and left-over food (brown beans preferred), one and one half tablespoonfuls vegetable butter, two teaspoonfuls chopped onion, a sprinkle of sage and marjoram, one tablespoonful brown flour, one third cup milk, one egg, and salt to taste. Soak the bread in cold water until soft all the way through; then press out lightly. Put the butter, the onion, and the savory into a small pan, and simmer for a few moments. Add the brown flour, then the milk, and stir until smooth. Mash the beans with a spoon, beat the egg slightly, and mix all the ingredients. Bake in an oiled baking pan until set, and brown on the top. Loosen with a knife along the edge, turn out on a platter, and serve.

Country Gravy. — Cook down a little sour cream in a pan until the oil separates and the albumen turns a very light brown color; then add enough flour (previously browned in the oven) to take up the fat from the cream. Add a little hot milk, and stir smooth. Add more milk, and bring to a boil and the thickness of medium thin gravy.

Stewed Corn. — Take cooked corn cut off the cob, add a little hot water, and bring to a boil. Season with a little cream or vegetable butter, reheat, and serve.

Fruit Soup. — Two cups blackberry or strawberry juice, four tablespoonfuls sago, two teaspoonfuls lemon juice, two cups water, sugar to taste. Wash the sago, drain, add to two cups boiling water, and let cook until clear. Add the fruit juices, and sweeten to taste. Preferably served cold.

Buckwheat Wafers. — This recipe follows the recipe given for buckwheat sticks in Thursday's lesson.

SATURDAY

Breakfast

CREAM HOMINY	GRAPEFRUIT	STEWED PRUNES
SOY TOAST	BUTTER	RYE BREAD

Dinner

LETTUCE	WHOLE RICE WITH NEW PEAS	COTTAGE CHEESE
SUMMER SQUASH	RAISIN PIE	ENTIRE WHEAT BREAD

Luncheon

FIGS	MILK TOAST	PEAR SAUCE
CREAM ROLLS		CEREAL COFFEE

Cream Hominy. — Heat a little cream, or a little milk and a small seasoning of vegetable butter. Add enough lye hominy to make the food creamy and not too milky. Add a pinch of salt, and serve.

Soy Toast. — Duplicate the recipe for cream peas on toast, as given in Sunday's breakfast lesson, substituting thoroughly cooked and mashed soy beans for the peas, and serve.

Whole Rice with Peas.—One half cup uncooked natural brown rice, one and one half cups boiling water, one and one half cups cooked new peas, one tablespoonful vegetable butter, two teaspoonfuls flour, salt. Wash the rice thoroughly, put to cook in one and one half cups boiling water, and let boil steadily until the water is evaporated and the rice looks dry; then cover, and let stand on the edge of the stove to steam for fifteen minutes. Add enough hot water to the peas to cover them, salt to season, and let cook gently until the liquid is reduced to one half cupful, and the peas are tender. Rub the flour and the butter together in a saucepan. Add a little of the liquid from the peas, and stir smooth. Add the balance of the liquid, and boil up. Add the peas to the rice, pour on the thin sauce, and mix with a fork. Put into a covered dish, and set into the oven until hot through.

Summer Squash.—Wash the squash, peel very thinly, remove the seeds if they are large, and steam the squash until tender. Mash, season with a little cream or vegetable butter, and serve.

Raisin Pie.—One and one half cupfuls seedless sultana raisins, two cupfuls water, one tablespoonful lemon juice, one scant tablespoonful cornstarch, one third cup sugar, one teaspoonful vegetable butter. Wash the raisins thoroughly, and soak overnight. Bring to a boil with the two cupfuls water; then add the sugar mixed with the starch, a pinch of salt, and let boil for about ten minutes, or until the liquid is reduced suitably for one pie. Let cool.

Pie Crust.—One and one fourth cups pastry flour, four tablespoonfuls solid vegetable fat, one eighth teaspoonful salt, about three tablespoonfuls water. Add the salt and the shortening to the flour, and mix with the finger tips. Add the water very slowly, mixing with a fork, as it runs in, to a soft, light dough. Line the bottom of a pie tin with crust, being careful to press the crust well down into the tin; then pour on the stewed raisins. Add the lemon juice and the vegetable butter; then cover with a perforated top crust, having the edges wet, so as to stick the crusts together. Brush over the top with milk, and bake in a quick oven.

Cream Rolls.—One and one third cups pastry flour, two thirds cup whole wheat flour, one half teaspoonful salt, one teaspoonful sugar, one third cup double cream, one fourth cup cold water. Mix the water and the cream thoroughly. Put all the dry ingredients into a bowl, and pour on the wetting in a very slow stream, stirring constantly, so as to get the moisture evenly blended through the flour. Work into a dough, roll out to about one half inch thickness, and cut into long strips about one third inch in width. Roll each piece on the board, and cut into three-inch lengths. Lay in a baking pan, leaving a little space between, and bake in a medium oven, to a light brown.

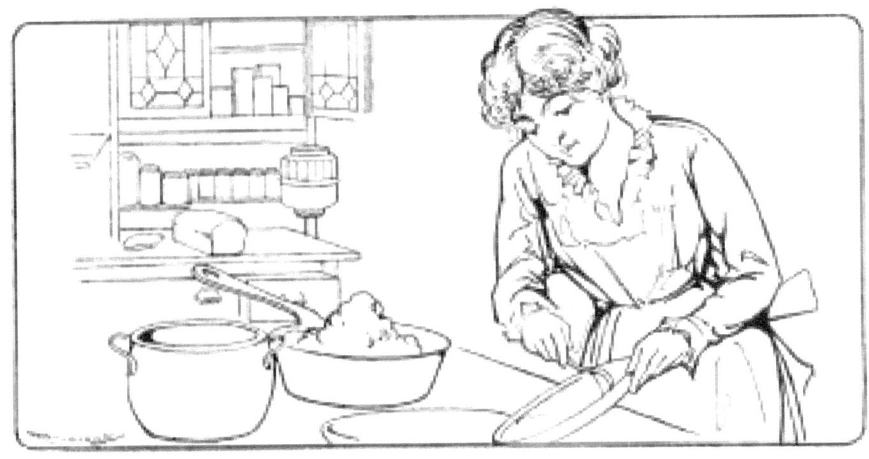

THE USE OF LEFT-OVERS

BY

DR. LAVINA BAXTER-HERZER

Department of Pathology and Bacteriology,
College of Medical Evangelists,
Loma Linda, California

At the present time, when the conservation of food is such a vital question, the use of left-overs becomes a very important matter for consideration. The following are a few simple suggestions that may prove helpful.

First of all, we should plan, as far as possible, to avoid having much food left. One of the simplest means of accomplishing this is to serve fewer foods at a meal. Variety may be had at different meals.

By planning beforehand, we can serve such foods at one meal as will combine nicely when warmed the next day or the next meal.

For example: In all large hotels, when navy bean soup is served army style, carrots are always served in some way. In order to make the broth sufficiently rich, more beans are cooked than are served as soup. The next day, these, with the carrots, are put through a soup strainer, properly seasoned, and served as puree a la Crecy.

Again, when planning tomato rice soup, cook a little extra rice in the tomato broth. When serving the soup, use only what rice is necessary. The thick remainder is very good baked in some acceptable preparation the next day. A little grated onion or a chopped bell pepper may be used for seasoning, if desired.

A Housewife's Test

After meals, the first thing that should claim the housewife's attention is the food that remains uneaten. Just here is one of the tests of her ability to do her part in conserving her family food supply. It is quicker, perhaps, to scrape everything into the garbage pail; and it is said that at least twenty per cent of all foods brought into American kitchens is lost in this way. This loss either decreases the amount of food the family should have, or raises the cost of living that much.

If food is to be kept over, it should be put into dishes of proper size, and put in a cool place, away from the flies and the dust. The sooner these left-overs are used, the better, as they naturally deteriorate by standing.

In case of fresh fruit, it may be heated, if there is any doubt as to its keeping.

Apple peelings and cores make excellent jelly, as most of the pectin is found near the skin and the seeds. Care should be taken to wash the apples well before paring, and remove any wormy parts.

All butter scraps should be saved, and may be used for cooking. If the family is properly taught, however, there will be very little left on the plates.

Left-over bread may be used for toast, bread pudding, or pressed fruit pudding, if unbroken. The broken pieces and the crumbs may be dried and used for dressing, or broken or rolled and served with milk instead of fresh bread.

Buns, muffins, and gems may be moistened and reheated. A loaf of very stale bread may be freshened in the same way.

Left-over vegetables may be reheated, and used for salad, or for flavoring soups, if put through a soup strainer.

Salads do not keep well; and for that reason, care should be taken not to prepare more than is likely to be eaten. If a little is left, it may be used for a pick-up lunch, perhaps. Small portions of dessert may be used in the same way.

Milk or cream that is left may be sterilized and put in a cool place.

Left-over grains may be used for making gruels, which are very good for lunch; or if only a small amount remains, it may be used for thickening soup. If there is a sufficient amount, steamed raisins or dates may be added, and then it may be put into molds to cool. This may be served with cream or some pudding sauce, making a simple dessert for either dinner or lunch. Cream of wheat, rolled wheat, farina, and Graham are especially nice served in this way.

Many housewives cook an extra amount of corn meal in order to have some left, as it is better warmed up than at the first. It is good mixed with croutons, rolled in corn flakes, browned, and served with jelly or maple sirup. To mix with rice or any nut food, season, form into patties, and serve with tomato sauce, is another method.

When warming potatoes, if the supply is scant, many persons add a slice of stale bread broken up.

The vegetable loaf given in Mr. Anderson's recipes may be varied, and any kind of beans or peas used to make it. Served with a good gravy, it makes a substantial dish for dinner.

By using a choux paste, left-over rice, macaroni, spaghetti, any kind of beans, peas, or lentils may be made into patties or croquettes. They may be served with gravy or jelly, and their original form scarcely be recognized when they appear on the table next time.

To make the choux paste, take one and one half tablespoons of butter, dairy or vegetable, one tablespoon of chopped onion, and a pinch of sage. Put in a small saucepan, and stir over the fire a few minutes, but do not brown. Add three tablespoons of flour, and stir until it is thoroughly scalded. Then add one third cup of milk, and stir until smooth. Drop into this mixture the yolk of one egg, and stir until it is well cooked. It should be a thick, smooth paste when done. Part of this may be used one day, and the rest saved for another time.

As the housewife seeks to make use of all remnants of food, new possibilities will gradually open before her, and her efforts will become a real pleasure rather than a task.

THE call is, therefore, to YOU to do your part; and in the doing, you will bind yourself to the whole army of women who are serving their country.

—Dr. Anna Howard Shaw.

Lector House believes that a society develops through a two-fold approach of continuous learning and adaptation, which is derived from the study of classic literary works spread across the historic timeline of literature records. Therefore, we aim at reviving, repairing and redeveloping all those inaccessible or damaged but historically as well as culturally important literature across subjects so that the future generations may have an opportunity to study and learn from past works to embark upon a journey of creating a better future.

This book is a result of an effort made by Lector House towards making a contribution to the preservation and repair of original ancient works which might hold historical significance to the approach of continuous learning across subjects.

HAPPY READING & LEARNING!

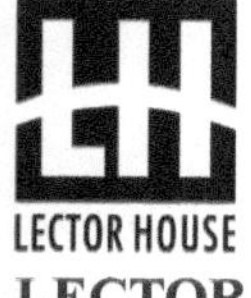

LECTOR HOUSE LLP
E-MAIL: lectorpublishing@gmail.com